I0484290

Evidence Synthesis
Number 115

Screening for Gonorrhea and Chlamydia: Systematic Review to Update the U.S. Preventive Services Task Force Recommendations

Prepared for:
Agency for Healthcare Research and Quality
U.S. Department of Health and Human Services
540 Gaither Road
Rockville, MD 20850
www.ahrq.gov

Contract No. HHS-290-2007-10057-I, Task Order No. 13

Prepared by:
Pacific Northwest Evidence-Based Practice Center
Oregon Health & Science University
3181 SW Sam Jackson Park Road
Portland, OR 97239
www.ohsu.edu/epc

Investigators:
Heidi D. Nelson, MD, MPH
Bernadette Zakher, MBBS
Amy Cantor, MD, MPH
Monica Deagas, BA
Miranda Pappas, MA

AHRQ Publication No. 13-05184-EF-1
September 2014

Acknowledgements

The authors acknowledge Andrew Hamilton, MLS, MS, at the Oregon Health & Science University; Karen Lee, MD, MPH, at AHRQ; and current and former members of the U.S. Preventive Services Task Force who contributed to topic deliberations.

Suggested Citation

Nelson HD, Zakher B, Cantor A, Deagas M, Pappas M. Screening for Gonorrhea and Chlamydia: Systematic Review to Update the U.S. Preventive Services Task Force Recommendations. Evidence Synthesis No. 115. AHRQ Publication No. 13-05184-EF-1. Rockville, MD: Agency for Healthcare Research and Quality; 2014.

Structured Abstract

Background: Previous research has supported screening for gonorrhea and chlamydia in asymptomatic sexually active women, including pregnant women, who are younger than age 25 years or at increased risk, but not other patient populations.

Purpose: To update the 2005 and 2007 systematic reviews for the U.S. Preventive Services Task Force on screening for gonorrhea and chlamydia in men and women, including pregnant women and adolescents.

Data Sources: MEDLINE (2004 to June 13, 2014), Cochrane Central Register of Controlled Trials (through May 2014), Cochrane Database of Systematic Reviews (through May 2014), Health Technology Assessment Database (through May 2014), Database of Abstracts of Reviews of Effects (through May 2014), and reference lists.

Study Selection: English-language trials and observational studies about screening effectiveness, test accuracy, and screening harms.

Data Extraction: One investigator extracted data on participants, study design, analysis, followup, and results and a second investigator confirmed key data. Investigators independently dual-rated study quality and applicability using established criteria.

Data Synthesis: Screening a subset of asymptomatic young women for chlamydia in a good-quality trial did not statistically significantly reduce pelvic inflammatory disease over the following year (relative risk, 0.39 [95% CI, 0.14 to 1.08]), while one previous trial reported a reduction. An observational study evaluating a risk prediction tool to identify persons with chlamydia in high-risk populations had low predictive ability and applicability. In 10 new studies of asymptomatic participants, nucleic acid amplification tests demonstrated sensitivity of 86% or greater and specificity of 97% or greater for diagnosing gonorrhea and chlamydia, regardless of specimen type or test.

Limitations: Studies of screening benefits and harms were lacking for men, pregnant women, adolescents, and subgroups. Only screening tests and methods cleared by the U.S. Food and Drug Administration for current clinical practice were included to determine diagnostic accuracy, excluding rectal, pharyngeal, and self-administered specimens obtained outside a clinical setting.

Conclusions: Chlamydia screening in young women may reduce pelvic inflammatory disease. Nucleic acid amplification tests are accurate for diagnosing gonorrhea and chlamydia in asymptomatic persons using various types of specimens. Research is needed on the effectiveness of screening to reduce adverse health outcomes in specific population groups, effectiveness of different screening strategies, and adverse effects of screening to further inform practice guidelines.

Table of Contents

Figures

Tables

Appendixes

CHAPTER 1. INTRODUCTION

Purpose and Previous U.S. Preventive Services Task Force Recommendation

This report will be used by the U.S. Preventive Services Task Force (USPSTF) to update its 2005 recommendation on screening for gonorrhea[1] and its 2007 recommendation on screening for chlamydia.[2] It focuses on studies published since prior USPSTF systematic reviews of these topics.[3-5] **Appendix A** provides a description of terms and abbreviations used in this report.

In 2005, the USPSTF issued a B recommendation to screen for gonorrhea in all sexually active women at increased risk for infection, including pregnant women.[1] Women at increased risk include those who are younger than age 25 years; live in high prevalence communities; have a history of gonococcal infection or other sexually transmitted infections (STIs); have new or multiple sex partners; or engage in inconsistent condom use, sex work, or drug use. The USPSTF recommended against routine screening in men and nonpregnant women at low risk for infection (D recommendation), and found insufficient evidence to recommend for or against routine screening in high-risk men and low-risk pregnant women (I statement).

In 2007, the USPSTF issued an A recommendation to screen for chlamydia in all sexually active nonpregnant women younger than age 25 years and in older high-risk nonpregnant women (i.e., those who have a history of chlamydial infection or other STIs, have new or multiple sex partners, or engage in inconsistent condom use or sex work).[2] The age specification for screening in the 2007 recommendation differed from the previous recommendation (age ≤25 years) in order to align with evidence on screening, including national surveillance data from the Centers for Disease Control and Prevention (CDC). The USPSTF also recommended screening in pregnant women younger than age 25 years and in older high-risk pregnant women (B recommendation), and recommended against routine screening in low-risk women age 25 years or older regardless of pregnancy status (C recommendation). The USPSTF found insufficient evidence to recommend for or against routine screening in men (I statement).

Condition Definition

Gonorrhea is an STI caused by the bacterium *Neisseria gonorrhoeae*, a gram-negative intracellular diplococcus that infects the mucosal epithelium of the genital tract.[6,7] Other sites of infection include the conjunctiva, oropharynx, and rectum. Infection with *N. gonorrhoeae* often leads to local inflammation and, in women, can ascend the urogenital tract and cause pelvic inflammatory disease (PID).[6] Infants born to infected mothers may contract gonococcal eye disease in the first few days of life.[8]

Chlamydia is an STI caused by the bacterium *Chlamydia trachomatis*. Most *C. trachomatis* strains infect the epithelial cells of the genital tract, causing inflammation that may be asymptomatic or present as erythema, edema, and mucopurulent discharge.[9] Infections of the rectum can cause proctitis, while infections of the oropharynx are typically asymptomatic. Inflammation damages the epithelium and leads to scar formation. In women, scarring may ultimately lead to fallopian tube occlusion and infertility years after active infection. Infants born to infected mothers may contract chlamydial eye disease and pneumonia.[8,9]

Prevalence

Gonorrhea is the second most commonly reported STI in the United States after chlamydia. In 2012, 334,826 cases were reported to the CDC, although less than half of all cases are actually diagnosed and reported.[10] Prevalence rates among women and men are similar (108.7 vs. 105.8 cases per 100,000, respectively), and the highest rates of infection are among persons ages 15 to 24 years.

Chlamydia is the most commonly reported STI in the United States. In 2012, 1,422,976 cases of chlamydia were reported to the CDC.[10] However, the true incidence of chlamydia is difficult to accurately estimate because most infections are asymptomatic and are therefore undetected. In 2012, the rate of chlamydial infection among women (643.3 cases per 100,000) was more than double the rate among men (262.6 cases per 100,000), with the majority of cases occurring among women ages 15 to 24 years.

Estimates of coinfection with both gonorrhea and chlamydia are not available.

Pregnancy

In 2011, CDC surveillance data indicated that the median State-specific gonorrhea positivity rate among women ages 15 to 24 years screened in selected prenatal clinics in 15 states, Puerto Rico, and the Virgin Islands was 0.8 percent (range, 0.0% to 3.8%), and the chlamydia positivity rate was 7.7 percent (range, 2.8% to 16.3%).[8] The risk for mother-to-child transmission of gonorrhea is between 30 and 47 percent.[11]

Etiology, Natural History, and Burden of Disease

Gonococcal infections in women are often asymptomatic, but can cause cervicitis and complications of PID, such as ectopic pregnancy, infertility, and chronic pelvic pain.[8] Gonorrhea in men can lead to symptomatic urethritis, epididymitis, and prostatitis.[12] The majority of urethral infections in men are symptomatic, resulting in timely treatment that prevents serious complications.[13] However, infections at extragenital sites (i.e., pharynx and rectum) are typically asymptomatic. Rarely, local gonococcal infections disseminate, causing an acute dermatitis tenosynovitis syndrome that can be complicated by arthritis, meningitis, or endocarditis.[7,14] Gonorrhea facilitates HIV transmission in both men and women.[8]

As with gonorrhea, chlamydial infections in women are usually asymptomatic, but can cause cervicitis and urethritis.[15] Ten to 15 percent of untreated chlamydial infections progress to symptomatic PID that can cause infertility, chronic pelvic pain, and ectopic pregnancy.[8,15]

Genital chlamydial infection in men is usually asymptomatic, but can cause nongonococcal urethritis, epididymitis, and, in rare instances, uretheral strictures and reactive arthritis.[8,16] Chlamydia can also infect nongenital sites and can facilitate the transmission of HIV infection.[8,17,18]

Risk Factors

Age is a strong predictor of risk for both gonorrhea and chlamydia. In 2012, rates of gonococcal infection reported to the CDC were highest among women ages 20 to 24 years (578.5 cases per 100,000), women ages 15 to 19 years (521.2 cases per 100,000), and men ages 20 to 24 years (462.8 cases per 100,000). Rates of chlamydial infection were also highest among women ages 20 to 24 years (3,695.5 cases per 100,000), women ages 15 to 19 years (3,291.5 cases per 100,000), and men ages 20 to 24 years (1,350.4 cases per 100,000).[10]

Infection rates vary by race and ethnicity. In 2012, rates of gonococcal infection among blacks (462.0 cases per 100,000), American Indians/Alaska Natives (124.9 cases per 100,000), Native Hawaiians/Other Pacific Islanders (87.8 cases per 100,000), and Hispanics (60.4 cases per 100,000) were higher than among whites (31.0 cases per 100,000) and Asians (16.9 cases per 100,000). The rates of chlamydial infection among blacks (1,229.4 cases per 100,000), American Indians/Alaska Natives (728.2 cases per 100,000), Native Hawaiians/Other Pacific Islanders (590.4 cases per 100,000), and Hispanics (380.3 cases per 100,000) were also higher than among whites (179.6 cases per 100,000) and Asians (112.9 cases per 100,000).[10]

Infection rates are high among specific population subgroups. Among men who have sex with men (MSM) tested at 42 STI clinics in 12 local and state health jurisdictions during 2012, the median gonorrhea prevalence rate was 16.4 percent (range, 9.8% to 30.4%), and the chlamydia prevalence rate was 12.0 percent (range, 6.4% to 22.2%).[10] Among men and women enrolled in the National Job Training Program, a program for socioeconomically disadvantaged youth ages 16 to 24 years, median prevalence rates for chlamydia in 2012 were 11.0 percent (range, 5.5% to 19.4%) in women and 7.0 percent (range, 0.6% to 13.5%) in men.[10] Prevalence rates for gonorrhea were 1.3 percent (range, 0.0% to 4.8%) in women and 0.7 percent (range, 0.0% to 2.8%) in men. Among adolescents entering selected juvenile correctional facilities in 2011, prevalence of gonorrhea ranged from 0.1 to 4.9 percent and from 5.4 to 17.3 percent for chlamydia.[8] Prevalence rates were generally higher among women than men for both infections.

Other risk factors include having new or multiple sex partners or a partner with an STI, inconsistent condom use, and history of previous or coexisting STIs.[3,4]

Rationale for Screening and Screening Strategies

Gonorrhea and chlamydia are often asymptomatic in infected women, but can cause serious complications[10] and be transmitted to sex partners and unborn children. Screening has the potential to improve the detection and treatment of infected individuals and reduce the severity of complications of untreated disease and transmission. The two infections have comparable distributions in populations and can be detected using similar tests from the same specimen. The availability of accurate screening tests and effective treatments make screening a feasible approach.

Interventions and Treatment

Infection with *N. gonorrhoeae* can be detected by nucleic acid amplification tests (NAATs) using male and female urine and clinician-collected endocervical, vaginal, and male urethral specimens.[10] Most NAATs cleared for use on clinician-collected vaginal swabs are also cleared for use on self-collected vaginal specimens obtained in clinical settings. Rectal and pharyngeal swabs can be collected from persons who engage in receptive anal and oral intercourse, although these sites of collection have not been cleared by the U.S. Food and Drug Administration (FDA). Gonorrhea can also be detected by culture, which is recommended for diagnosing resistant strains and for detecting strains with decreased antimicrobial susceptibility. Antimicrobial susceptibility testing can only be performed using culture.

Current recommendations support using NAATs to detect *C. trachomatis* infections because their sensitivity and specificity are high and they have been cleared by the FDA for use on urogenital sites, including male and female urine, as well as clinician-collected endocervical, vaginal, and male urethral specimens.[10] Most NAATs cleared for use on vaginal swabs are also cleared for use on self-collected vaginal specimens obtained in clinical settings. Rectal swabs can be collected from persons who engage in receptive anal intercourse, although this site of collection has not been cleared by the FDA.

Gonorrhea and chlamydia respond to antibiotic treatment. In recent years, treatment of gonorrhea has been complicated by increasing drug resistance. For nonpregnant adults, new recommendations have replaced the use of oral cephalosporins with a single intramuscular dose of ceftriaxone in combination with either single-dose azithromycin or 7-day doxycycline for the treatment of uncomplicated gonorrhea of the cervix, urethra, and rectum.[19] Combination therapy is recommended to prevent the development of further drug resistance, as well as to treat commonly coexisting chlamydia. Azithromycin is generally preferred to doxycycline as the secondary drug in gonorrhea combination treatment because of its convenience as a single-dose therapy, as well as evidence of gonorrhea resistance to tetracyclines such as doxycycline. Chlamydia is treated with single-dose azithromycin or 7-day doxycycline.[13] In patients for whom adherence or followup is a concern, azithromycin is the preferred choice because it provides a single dose of directly observed treatment.

For patients with either gonorrhea or chlamydia, all sex partners from the preceding 60 days should be evaluated and treated for infection.[13,15,19] Expedited partner therapy is a means of treatment in which medication or a prescription is delivered to the partner by the patient, a disease investigation specialist, or a pharmacy.[19] In the case of treatment for gonorrhea, the partner would receive oral combination therapy with cefixime and azithromycin, rather than intramuscular ceftriaxone. All patients diagnosed with gonorrhea or chlamydia require retesting 3 months after treatment.[13,15]

Pregnancy

Pregnant women infected with gonorrhea require intramuscular ceftriaxone and oral azithromycin.[10,13] Chlamydial infections in pregnant women are treated with single-dose azithromycin or 7-day amoxicillin.[13] In addition, a test of cure to document eradication of chlamydial infection 3 weeks after treatment is recommended. Pregnant women diagnosed with chlamydia or gonorrhea in the first trimester should also be retested 3 months after treatment. Gonococcal neonatal ophthalmia, resulting from transmission from an untreated woman to her newborn, may be prevented with routine topical prophylaxis at delivery. However, prevention of chlamydial neonatal pneumonia and ophthalmia require prenatal detection and treatment.

Current Clinical Practice

Despite current guidelines that recommend screening for gonorrhea and chlamydia in high-risk persons, a review of the health care claims of 4,296 men and women presenting for general medical or gynecological examinations from 2000 to 2003 found that almost none had codes for screening for HIV, syphilis, gonorrhea, or chlamydia, regardless of their high-risk sexual behavior status.[20] Among patients claiming high-risk sexual behaviors, only 21 to 56 percent were tested for gonorrhea and 21 to 60 percent were tested for chlamydia. Similarly, a review of the U.S. Healthcare Effectiveness Data and Information Set from 2000 to 2007 showed a 64.4 percent increase in testing for chlamydia among young, sexually active women enrolled in commercial and Medicaid health plans during that period; however, the testing rate in 2007 was only 41.6 percent.[21] Population-based survey data from 2005 to 2008 in the United States indicated that many pregnant women were not tested, and followup testing was not always performed.[22]

Recommendations of Other Groups

The CDC's recommendations are similar to those of the USPSTF and include targeted screening for gonorrhea and chlamydia in women at increased risk, while screening in other groups, including men, is not recommended.[1,2,13] The CDC also advises screening in other selected high-risk populations, including MSM and young women in juvenile detention or jail facilities. Recommendations from the CDC and other professional groups are summarized in **Table 1**.

CHAPTER 2. METHODS

Key Questions and Analytic Framework

This review followed a standard protocol consistent with the Agency for Healthcare Research and Quality's (AHRQ's) methods for systematic reviews.[23,24] Based on evidence gaps identified from prior reviews,[3-5] the USPSTF and AHRQ determined the scope and Key Questions of the review. A research plan was externally reviewed and modified. Investigators created two analytic frameworks incorporating the Key Questions and outlining the patient populations, interventions, outcomes, and potential adverse effects. The first analytic framework is for asymptomatic, sexually active men and nonpregnant women, including adolescents (**Figure 1**). The second analytic framework is for pregnant women (**Figure 2**).

The review includes studies published since prior USPSTF reviews of these topics.[3-5] Studies were included if they were applicable to clinical settings and practices in the United States, as determined by the similarity of participants and health care services to real-world situations and the use of screening tests that are available and FDA-cleared for clinical use. The conditions of interest are gonococcal and chlamydial infections in asymptomatic persons.

The Key Questions for men and nonpregnant women are:

1. How effective is screening for gonorrhea and chlamydia in reducing complications of infection and transmission or acquisition of disease in asymptomatic, sexually active men and nonpregnant women, including adolescents?
2. How effective are different screening strategies in identifying persons with gonorrhea and chlamydia?
3. How accurate are screening tests in detecting gonorrhea and chlamydia?
4. What are the harms of screening for gonorrhea and chlamydia?

The Key Questions for pregnant women are:

1. How effective is screening for gonorrhea and chlamydia in reducing maternal complications, adverse pregnancy and infant outcomes, and transmission or acquisition of disease in asymptomatic pregnant women?
2. What are the harms of screening for gonorrhea and chlamydia in asymptomatic pregnant women?

Search Strategies

The investigators worked with a research librarian to conduct searches of electronic databases, including MEDLINE (2004 to June 13, 2014), Cochrane Central Register of Controlled Trials (through May 2014), Cochrane Database of Systematic Reviews (through May 2014), Health Technology Assessment Database (through May 2014), Database of Abstracts of Reviews of Effects (through May 2014), and clinicaltrials.gov (through May 2014) (search strategies are available in **Appendix B1**). Search dates were selected to update prior USPSTF systematic reviews of these topics. In addition, investigators manually reviewed reference lists of relevant articles.

Study Selection

Abstracts were selected for full-text review if they included asymptomatic, sexually active men and women, including pregnant women and adolescents; were relevant to a Key Question; and met additional prespecified inclusion criteria for each Key Question. Although this update was intended to evaluate studies published since prior USPSTF reviews, the scope, Key Questions, and inclusion criteria differ across reviews, resulting in the inclusion of some apparently older studies that had not been previously reviewed. Two reviewers independently evaluated each study to determine its inclusion eligibility based on prespecified inclusion and exclusion criteria developed for each Key Question (**Appendix B2**). Non-English–language articles and studies published as abstracts were not included.

Studies of screening effectiveness (Key Questions 1 and 2 for general populations and Key Question 1 for pregnant women) were included if they compared health outcomes of screened and nonscreened asymptomatic persons. Outcomes included reduced complications of gonococcal or chlamydial infections and reduced transmission or acquisition of disease, and for pregnant women, reduced maternal complications, adverse pregnancy outcomes, and adverse infant outcomes. Only randomized, controlled trials (RCTs) and controlled observational studies were included to evaluate the effectiveness of screening. Studies of screening strategies were included if they described the study population (number screened, sex, age range, setting, and absence of symptoms), features of the screening program (duration, type of strategy, and followup), and outcome measures. Inclusion criteria for effectiveness studies were less restrictive than for diagnostic accuracy studies because the main comparison concerned outcomes related to the overall approach of screening versus not screening, not the individual tests themselves. Uncontrolled observational studies were included to determine adverse effects of screening (Key Question 4 for general populations and Key Question 2 for pregnant women).

Studies of diagnostic accuracy (Key Question 3) were included if they evaluated the performance of tests in asymptomatic persons using technologies and methods cleared by the FDA and available for clinical practice in the United States. Based on these criteria, rectal, pharyngeal, and self-collected vaginal specimens obtained in nonclinical settings, as well as point-of-care or in-house tests, were excluded. Tests that were previously cleared by the FDA and subsequently removed from the U.S. market were also excluded.[25] Included studies of diagnostic accuracy used credible reference standards, described the study population (number screened, sex, age range, setting, and absence of symptoms), defined positive screening test results, and reported performance characteristics (sensitivity, specificity, positive and negative predictive values, positive and negative likelihood ratios) or provided data to calculate them.

The selection of studies is summarized in **Appendix B3**. **Appendix B4** lists studies excluded at the full-text level with reasons for exclusion.

Data Abstraction and Quality Rating

One investigator abstracted details about study design, patient population, comparison groups, setting, screening method, analysis, followup, and results. A second investigator reviewed data abstraction for accuracy. By using prespecified criteria developed by the USPSTF for RCTs, cohort, and diagnostic accuracy studies,[24] two investigators independently rated the quality of studies (good, fair, or poor) and resolved discrepancies by consensus (**Appendix B5**).

Data Synthesis

Two independent reviewers assessed the internal validity (quality) of new studies for each Key Question using methods developed by the USPSTF, based on the number, quality, and size of studies; consistency of results between studies; and directness of evidence.[23,24] Statistical meta-analysis was not performed because of methodological limitations of the studies and heterogeneity in study designs, interventions, populations, and other factors. Studies included in prior reviews were reviewed for consistency with current results; however, lack of studies and differences in scope, Key Questions, and inclusion criteria limited aggregate synthesis with the updated evidence.

External Review

The draft report was reviewed by six content experts and scientists at the CDC during October 2013 and by USPSTF members, AHRQ Project Officers, collaborative partners, and the public during May 2014 (**Appendix B6**).

Response to Public Comments

This systematic review was posted for public comment from April 29 to May 26, 2014. The investigators reviewed and considered relevant comments. No comments identified missing studies that met inclusion criteria or errors in the evidence reviewed, resulting in no changes to the findings or the conclusion of this report.

CHAPTER 3. RESULTS

Men and Nonpregnant Women, Including Adolescents

Key Question 1. How Effective Is Screening for Gonorrhea and Chlamydia in Reducing Complications of Infection and Transmission or Acquisition of Disease in Asymptomatic, Sexually Active Men and Nonpregnant Women, Including Adolescents?

Summary

No studies of screening for gonorrhea met inclusion criteria for the prior USPSTF reviews or this update. One study of the effectiveness of screening for chlamydia met inclusion criteria. The Prevention of Pelvic Infection (POPI) trial reported a nonstatistically significant reduction in incident PID among asymptomatic, sexually active young women screened for chlamydia compared with unscreened women (relative risk [RR], 0.39 [95% CI, 0.14 to 1.08])[26] (S Kerry, written communication, May 2013).

The 2001[3] and 2007[5] USPSTF reviews on screening for chlamydia identified two trials of screening in women at increased risk for chlamydia (**Table 2** and **Appendix C1**).[27,28] PID was statistically significantly reduced among women screened in a good-quality RCT of young women recruited from a health maintenance organization in the United States (RR, 0.44 [95% CI, 0.20 to 0.90]).[27,28] Reductions were of borderline statistical significance in a poor-quality RCT of Danish students (RR, 0.50 [95% CI, 0.23 to 1.08]).[27,28]

Evidence

Gonorrhea. No effectiveness studies of screening for gonorrhea met inclusion criteria for this update or for prior USPSTF reviews.

Chlamydia. One new RCT of screening for chlamydia in women, but none in men, met inclusion criteria for this update. The POPI trial was a good-quality RCT of 2,529 sexually active young women (mean age, 21 years [range, 16 to 27 years]) recruited from universities and colleges in the United Kingdom (**Appendixes C1** and **C2**).[26] Participants were randomized to screening or deferred groups (considered unscreened), completed questionnaires, and provided self-collected vaginal swabs. Swabs from the screening group were immediately tested for chlamydia, while those from the deferred group were stored and tested 1 year later. Infected women were contacted and referred to their local clinic for treatment and partner notification. After 1 year, participants completed questionnaires about symptoms of PID and sexual behavior during the previous year (94% followup overall). Medical records of women suspected of having PID based on their questionnaire responses were obtained and reviewed by three blinded genitourinary physicians for diagnostic confirmation.

The published results of the trial provided RR estimates for developing PID during followup for symptomatic (35%) and asymptomatic (65%) participants combined (RR, 0.65 [95% CI, 0.34 to 1.22]).[26] Since asymptomatic women are the focus of this Key Question, the trial investigators provided additional estimates for this subgroup upon request. Among a subgroup of participants who reported no symptoms during the 6 months before the study (i.e., pelvic pain, dyspareunia, abnormal vaginal bleeding or discharge), 0.6 percent (5/787) of the screened group versus 1.6 percent (14/861) of the control group developed PID during followup (RR, 0.39 [95% CI, 0.14 to 1.08]) (S Kerry, written communication, May 2013).

In this trial, 79 percent (30/38) of PID cases overall occurred in women who tested negative at baseline. In addition, 22 percent of participants were tested for chlamydia independently during followup (23% and 22% of the screened and deferred groups, respectively). More women in the deferred group who tested positive for chlamydia had independent testing versus those who tested negative.

The 2001[3] and 2007[5] USPSTF reviews on screening for chlamydia identified two trials of the effectiveness of screening for prevention of PID in nonpregnant women (**Table 2**). A good-quality RCT of 2,607 women at increased risk for chlamydia in a health maintenance organization in Washington state reported a statistically significant reduction in PID in the screened versus usual care group after 1 year of followup (RR, 0.44 [95% CI, 0.20 to 0.90]).[27] In this trial, women randomized to screening were tested in study clinics. A poor-quality RCT of 1,761 female high school students in Denmark found that one-time, home-based screening compared with usual care (opportunistic physician-based screening) was associated with lower incidence of chlamydia (RR, 0.45 [95% CI, 0.24 to 0.84]) and PID (RR, 0.50 [95% CI, 0.23 to 1.08]) after 1 year of followup.[28] Since few participants were actually screened in the usual care group, they were considered to be similar to an unscreened comparison group.

Key Question 2. How Effective Are Different Screening Strategies in Identifying Persons With Gonorrhea and Chlamydia?

Summary

No studies compared the effectiveness of different screening strategies for gonorrhea or chlamydia in asymptomatic persons or the effectiveness of sampling from various anatomical sites, cotesting for concurrent STIs, or using different screening intervals. Several studies of screening in high-risk groups have been published, but they did not meet inclusion criteria because they enrolled both symptomatic and asymptomatic persons, lacked comparison groups, or did not report relevant outcomes. An observational study in the Netherlands evaluated a risk prediction tool to identify persons with chlamydia in high-risk populations.[29] However, the tool was not an accurate predictor, and its applicability to practice in the United States is unclear. Prior reviews did not directly address the effectiveness of different screening strategies, but rather summarized risk factors associated with gonococcal and chlamydial infections.[3,4] An observational study comparing nine sets of selective screening criteria for chlamydial infection among women attending family planning and STI clinics in the United States[30] indicated that age alone had similar or better sensitivity and specificity as more extensive criteria. In this study, nearly 80 percent of cases were identified when testing 50 percent of the population and using an age cutoff of 22 years or younger.

Evidence

An observational study conducted in the Netherlands evaluated a risk prediction tool to identify persons with chlamydia in high-risk populations (**Appendixes C3** and **C4**).[29] Screening criteria were developed on the basis of questionnaire responses from sexually active participants who were subsequently tested for chlamydia and included items on age, education, ethnicity, lifetime sex partners, and condom use. When applied to two high-risk populations, this risk tool was not an accurate predictor of infection (area under the receiver operating curve, 0.66 and 0.68, respectively). The applicability of this study to U.S. populations is also limited.

Key Question 3. How Accurate Are Screening Tests for Detecting Gonorrhea and Chlamydia?

Summary

Ten new fair-quality diagnostic accuracy studies reporting test characteristics of FDA-cleared NAATs met inclusion criteria, including six for gonorrhea and eight for chlamydia. Most studies evaluated the performance characteristics of NAATs compared with culture or expanded reference standards in asymptomatic persons in high prevalence (>5%) settings. Studies reporting the lowest values had important methodological limitations.

For gonorrhea, test sensitivity ranged from 90 to 100 percent in studies without major limitations, and specificity was greater than 97 percent across all specimens and tests. For chlamydia, test sensitivity ranged from 86 to 100 percent in studies without major limitations, and specificity was greater than 97 percent across all specimens and tests. In women, NAATs showed little variation across endocervical, clinician- and self-collected vaginal, and urine specimens. In men, urine specimens had slightly higher sensitivity than urethral specimens.

The prior reviews reported similar findings, but included several studies of non-NAAT tests, including some that are not currently available, as well as studies of symptomatic persons.[3,4]

Evidence

This review focused on the performance characteristics of screening tests in asymptomatic persons compared with either culture or expanded reference standards (i.e., positive result on two nonculture tests, positive result on two different specimens, or positive result on the original test and a confirmatory test). These studies included only FDA-cleared tests and specimen types (**Table 3**).

Ten new fair-quality studies reporting test characteristics of FDA-cleared NAATs met inclusion criteria, including six for gonorrhea (**Appendix C5**)[31-36] and eight for chlamydia (**Appendix C6**).[31-33,36-40] Methodological limitations include unclear descriptions of sampling methods, whether screening tests were interpreted independent of the reference standard,[31-34,37-39] and whether analyses included patients with uninterpretable results (**Appendix C7**).[31,33,34,37,39] Three studies described additional methodological difficulties related to the reference standard[38] and technical approach.[34,37] Most studies reported an infection prevalence of greater than 5 percent among participants, although rates were lower in three studies.[33,35,36]

Gonorrhea. Test characteristics of NAATs for gonorrhea are provided in **Table 4** for women and **Table 5** for men. All but three studies[33,35,36] reported an infection prevalence of greater than 5 percent among participants. Specificity was high (≥97%) across all studies for men and women regardless of specimen or test.

For women, four studies testing endocervical specimens with transcription mediated amplification (TMA); polymerase chain reaction (PCR), including a new rapid test;[36] or strand displacement amplification (SDA) reported sensitivities ranging from 90 to 100 percent (**Table 6** and **Figure 3**).[33-36] Sensitivity was 98 percent for TMA[35] and 100 percent for PCR[36] using self-collected vaginal specimens obtained in a clinician's office. Results for TMA, PCR, or SDA ranged from 78.6 to 100.0 percent using female urine.[33,34,36] However, the study reporting the lowest sensitivity used urine volumes larger than recommended by the manufacturer of the screening test.[34] When recommended urine volumes were used in a second study, the sensitivity of the same TMA test improved from 78.6 to 95.7 percent.[33]

For men, testing male urethral specimens with SDA and TMA and testing male urine with TMA, SDA, or PCR resulted in similarly high sensitivities across tests in four studies (urethra, 100%; urine, 90% to 100%) (**Table 6** and **Figure 3**).[31,32,34,36]

The 2005 evidence review on screening for gonorrhea reported sensitivity of 90 percent or greater and specificity of 97 percent or greater when cervical specimens were tested with NAATs or nucleic acid hybridization tests.[4] Testing female urine samples with PCR, TMA, or SDA had lower sensitivity (64.8% to 100.0%) than testing cervical specimens, although specificity was high across all specimens and tests. Male urine samples tested with PCR had lower sensitivity than testing urethral specimens, although this difference was not seen with SDA, and specificity was similar between specimen types for both tests. Many of these studies were conducted in high-prevalence populations and included both symptomatic and asymptomatic persons; few reported results by symptom status.

Chlamydia. Test characteristics of NAATs for chlamydia are provided in **Table 7** for women and **Table 8** for men. All but one study[36] reported greater than 5 percent prevalence of infection among participants. Specificity was high (≥96%) across all studies for men and women regardless of specimen or test.

Five studies of endocervical specimens reported sensitivity of TMA ranging from 89.0 to 97.1 percent, sensitivity of SDA ranging from 86.4 to 96.2 percent, and sensitivity of PCR ranging from 86.4 to 95.8 percent (**Table 6** and **Figure 4**).[33,36,37,39,40] Testing clinician-collected vaginal swabs with TMA or PCR resulted in sensitivities of 89.9 and 98.8 percent,[37] respectively, and testing self-collected vaginal swabs obtained in clinical settings resulted in sensitivities of 97.0 percent with TMA[40] and 90.7[37] and 98.0 percent[36] with PCR. Testing female urine samples with TMA, PCR, and SDA resulted in sensitivities ranging from 72.0 to 98.2 percent.[33,36,37,39] Lower sensitivities for testing urine samples with TMA (72%) and PCR (84%) were reported in one study that experienced technical and specimen processing errors.[37]

One study using PCR reported sensitivities that were markedly lower than those in other studies (endocervical, 51.9%; urine, 44.4%; clinician-collected vaginal, 55.6%; self-collected vaginal, 51.9%).[38] This study used a more conservative approach to analysis that only included women with complete sets of results from nine different testing strategies. In addition, the reference standard included positive NAAT results from two separate specimens. When a specimen-specific reference standard was used, as was common in the other studies, sensitivities were comparable with those in other studies (data not provided). Since these data represent outliers resulting from a different method, they are not included in **Figure 4**.

Sensitivities of testing male urethral and urine specimens with TMA, SDA, or PCR were consistently high across four studies, regardless of test, and ranged from 86.1 to 100.0 percent (**Figure 5**).[31,32,36,39]

The 2001 evidence review on screening for chlamydia found that testing endocervical swabs with enzyme immunoassay yielded lower sensitivity (70% to 80%) than PCR (82% to 100%), although specificity was similarly high (≥96%).[3] Testing urine with PCR performed comparably with testing endocervical swabs, and TMA was comparable with PCR. Testing male swab specimens with enzyme immunoassay had an average sensitivity of 80 percent and specificity of 96 to 100 percent, and testing with PCR resulted in higher sensitivity and specificity compared with enzyme immunoassay, similar to results for female specimens. Testing either male swab specimens or urine with PCR or TMA gave comparable performance results. Studies were conducted in high-prevalence populations and combined asymptomatic and symptomatic persons.

Key Question 4. What Are the Harms of Screening for Gonorrhea and Chlamydia?

Summary

New diagnostic accuracy studies without major methodological limitations indicated that false-positive rates for gonorrhea and chlamydia were 3 percent or less, and false-negative rates ranged from 0 to 9 percent for gonorrhea and 0 to 14 percent for chlamydia across all NAATs and specimen types. These results are consistent with prior reviews.[3-5] Several studies of psychosocial harms related to testing, such as anxiety, have been published, but did not meet inclusion criteria because they included symptomatic persons and focused on reactions to positive test results rather than screening itself.

A prior review[5] included results of qualitative interviews about the experience of chlamydia testing from women undergoing opportunistic screening.[41] Although many women felt that screening was beneficial and important, common responses to a positive test result included feeling dirty, ashamed at passing on the infection, and suspicious about the origins of the infection.

Evidence

Gonorrhea. Study results of screening tests for gonorrhea are provided in **Table 4** for women and **Table 5** for men. False-positive results were uniformly low across studies regardless of test or specimen, ranging from 0 to 2.9 percent. False-negative results had a wider range from 0 to 21.4 percent, although the highest rates can be attributed to studies with important methodological limitations (described previously).

No studies that addressed other harms, such as labeling or anxiety from screening, met inclusion criteria. The 2005 evidence review on screening for gonorrhea indicated similar findings for false-positive and false-negative results and did not address other harms of screening.[4]

Chlamydia. Study results of screening tests for chlamydia are provided in **Table 7** for women and **Table 8** for men. False-positive results were low across all studies regardless of specimen or test, ranging from 0 to 3.6 percent. Most studies of NAATs reported false-negative findings ranging from 0 to 28 percent, although the highest rates can be attributed to studies with important methodological limitations (described previously).[37,38] No studies that addressed other harms, such as labeling or anxiety from screening, met inclusion criteria.

The performance characteristics of chlamydia tests were evaluated in the 2001 review and were similar to this update, although the 2001 review included more studies of non-NAATs. The 2001[3] and 2007 reviews[5] identified no studies of harms of screening for chlamydia, but the more recent review contextually described three qualitative studies of the impact of receiving a positive chlamydia test result.

Pregnant Women

Key Question 1. How Effective Is Screening for Gonorrhea and Chlamydia in Reducing Complications of Infection and Transmission or Acquisition of Disease in Asymptomatic Pregnant Women?

No studies met inclusion criteria for this review as well as for the 2005 review on gonorrhea[4] and the 2007 review on chlamydia.[5] The 2001 review on chlamydia described a time-series and a case-control study predating the review conducted in the 1980s, but identified no new relevant studies.[3]

Key Question 2. What Are the Harms of Screening for Gonorrhea and Chlamydia in Asymptomatic Pregnant Women?

No studies met inclusion criteria, although the rates of false-positive and false-negative results for nonpregnant women are applicable to pregnant women. The prior reviews did not identify any relevant studies.

CHAPTER 4. DISCUSSION

Summary of Review Findings

The USPSTF and other groups currently recommend routine screening for gonorrhea and chlamydia in asymptomatic, sexually active women at increased risk for infection because of age or other risk factors, which is the standard of practice in the United States.[1,2,13,14,42-46] Previous recommendations were based on various levels of evidence indicating that screening provides an opportunity for earlier identification and treatment of infections and reduces adverse health outcomes and transmission.

A summary of evidence for this update is provided in **Table 9**. Only one new trial of the effectiveness of screening for chlamydia in nonpregnant women,[26] one study of a risk prediction instrument,[29] and 10 studies of the diagnostic accuracy of screening tests met inclusion criteria.[31-35,37-40] No studies were available to address several Key Questions. These include the effectiveness of screening for gonorrhea in all population groups and for chlamydia in men, pregnant women, and adolescents; the effectiveness of different screening strategies for identifying persons at increased risk for infection, cotesting for concurrent STIs, and different screening intervals; and harms of screening unrelated to the diagnostic accuracy of tests.

Only one new trial evaluated the effectiveness of screening for chlamydia in nonpregnant women[26] (Key Question 1). In the POPI trial, screening for chlamydia in a subset of asymptomatic young women did not statistically significantly reduce PID over the following year compared with not screening (RR, 0.39 [95% CI, 0.14 to 1.08]). Although it met criteria for good quality, the POPI trial was limited by inadequate recruitment, testing for chlamydia outside of the study protocol during followup in nearly a quarter of participants, and difficulty in ascertaining PID cases. These limitations imply that the study may have been underpowered and the intervention effects attenuated. In addition, most cases of PID occurred in women who tested negative at baseline, suggesting that frequent targeted screening in women at higher risk for infection, including those with new sex partners or recent history of chlamydia, might be more important than one-time routine screening.

Two earlier trials also evaluated incident PID after screening for chlamydia in women at increased risk.[27,28] While a good-quality trial in the United States reported a statistically significant reduction in PID in the screened versus usual care group after 1 year of followup (RR, 0.44 [95% CI, 0.20 to 0.90]),[27,28] reduction in PID was not statistically significant in a poor-quality trial in Denmark comparing one-time, home-based screening with usual care.[27,28] Although all three trials reported point estimates suggesting reduced PID, only the U.S. trial showed a statistically significant reduction. However, this trial met criteria for good quality, was the largest trial, and was the most applicable to clinical practice in the United States.

Additional relevant studies of screening did not meet inclusion criteria because they did not provide results for asymptomatic participants or reported infection rates rather than health outcomes. These studies found no significant improvements in clinical outcomes among those screened for chlamydia, including a large Danish trial of more than 30,000 young men and women,[47] a retrospective population-based cohort study of more than 40,000 Swedish women,[48] and a register-based screening trial of more than 300,000 men and women in the Netherlands.[49] A time-trend analysis of a U.S. managed care population between 1997 and 2007 indicated an increase in the number of cases of chlamydia in both men and women, but a decrease in PID.[50] It is not clear how screening influenced these outcomes.

The only new study addressing the effectiveness of different screening strategies (Key Question 2) was an observational study evaluating a risk prediction tool to identify persons with chlamydia in high-risk populations.[29] However, it was not an accurate predictor and its relevance to current practice in the United States is uncertain. An older observational study comparing nine sets of selective screening criteria for chlamydial infection among women[30] supports age-based screening in current guidelines, but has not been updated by newer research. Future studies to address this Key Question should compare the effectiveness of screening versus not screening in populations with different levels of risk; use specimens from different anatomical sites; include cotesting for concurrent STIs, including HIV; and evaluate different screening intervals.

Ten studies of the diagnostic accuracy of screening tests met inclusion criteria (Key Question 3).[31-35,37-40,51] The current review differs from prior reviews[3,4] by including only results from asymptomatic participants, which is more clinically relevant to screening populations. Various types of NAATs are highly accurate in diagnosing gonorrhea and chlamydia in asymptomatic persons regardless of specimen, anatomical site, or test.[31-34,37,39,51] Sensitivity was 85 percent or greater and specificity was 97 percent or greater in studies without major methodological limitations, resulting in generally low rates of false-negative and false-positive results. The high accuracy of NAATs reported in these studies is consistent with prior reviews[3,4] and is the basis for the CDC's recommendation on using NAATs for gonorrhea and chlamydia screening.[10]

Several studies of harms (Key Question 4) did not meet inclusion criteria for the update because they focused on the effects of receiving a positive test result, included symptomatic participants, and lacked comparison groups.[52-55] In these studies, persons who tested positive for chlamydia had higher measures of anxiety[52,53,55] and more partner break-ups[52,53] than those who tested negative, who were generally relieved.[53,55]

No studies addressing screening in pregnant women met inclusion criteria, despite the need for additional research in this population. For example, screening in the first trimester may not be sufficient based on findings from an observational study suggesting that chlamydia test results in the first trimester may not predict chlamydia status during the third trimester.[56] Although studies of repeat testing have been conducted in high-risk populations,[57] more research is warranted to further evaluate the value of repeat testing during pregnancy to reduce potential complications, such as preterm delivery and premature rupture of membranes.[58]

Limitations of this review include using only English-language articles, which could result in language bias, though we did not identify non-English–language studies otherwise meeting inclusion criteria in our searches. We only included studies with asymptomatic participants and settings and tests applicable to current practice in the United States to improve clinical relevance for the USPSTF, which excluded much research in the field. Studies were lacking for most Key Questions, and the number, quality, and applicability of studies varied widely. Available screening trials evaluated only PID as the main outcome, while other outcomes are also important.

NAATs are cleared by the FDA for use on male and female urine, endocervical, and male urethral specimens, and some types of NAATs are cleared for use on clinician- and self-collected vaginal specimens in clinical settings. Studies have also reported comparable test characteristics for nurse- and patient-collected rectal swabs in MSM.[35,37,38,40,59] Additional studies of NAATs using self-collected specimens could provide more evidence for FDA clearance of this technique and increase testing access and acceptability, potentially expanding screening strategies to home-, mail-, or Internet-based screening and encouraging uptake of screening among persons at increased risk.

Limiting our review to FDA-cleared tests excluded studies of rectal and pharyngeal specimens that also demonstrated high accuracy with NAATs,[35,37,38,40,59] which are currently recommended by the CDC.[10] Expanding the range of specimen types for screening has the potential to increase identification of infected persons, especially asymptomatic MSM, in whom nearly 90 percent of all gonococcal infections are at nongenital sites.[60] In this population, NAATs have higher sensitivity at extragenital sites compared with culture, possibly because of lower bacterial loads at the pharynx and rectum.[61,62] In a study of MSM, 85 percent of rectal infections were asymptomatic and only detectable with routine screening.[63] Urethral testing alone missed 84 percent of chlamydial and gonococcal infections compared with 9.8 percent missed by rectal and pharyngeal testing in another study.[60]

In summary, screening for chlamydia may reduce the incidence of PID in young women. Risk prediction tools may be useful in identifying persons with infections, but require validation in the populations of intended use. NAATs are accurate for diagnosing gonorrhea and chlamydia in asymptomatic persons regardless of specimen, anatomical site, or test. Further research is needed to determine the effectiveness of screening in multiple populations and on various clinical outcomes, including but not limited to PID, effective screening strategies, and harms of screening.

Limitations

The review included only English-language articles published since prior USPSTF reviews and does not reflect the total body of evidence on screening for gonorrhea and chlamydia, although relevant earlier studies were referenced. Studies were lacking for most Key Questions, and the number, quality, and applicability of studies varied widely.

This review explicitly focused on asymptomatic populations and included settings and tests applicable to current practice in the United States. While this approach improves its relevance to the USPSTF, it excludes much research in the field. For example, limiting the review to only FDA-cleared tests excluded studies of rectal and throat specimens that also demonstrated high accuracy with NAATs[35,37,38,40,59] and are currently used in practice. This is especially important for screening in asymptomatic MSM, in whom nearly 90 percent of all gonococcal infections are at nongenital sites (throat and rectum).[60]

Emerging Issues and Next Steps

Screening tests for gonorrhea and chlamydia accurately detect infections. In particular, the sensitivity of NAATs has surpassed culture, the former gold standard. NAATs have been cleared by the FDA for use on male and female urine, endocervical, and male urethral specimens, and some types of NAATs are cleared for use on clinician- and self-collected (in clinical settings) vaginal specimens. Studies have also reported comparable test characteristics for nurse- and patient-collected rectal swabs in MSM.[35,37,38,40,59] Additional studies of NAATs using self-collected specimens at various anatomical sites could provide more evidence for FDA clearance of this technique and increase testing access and acceptability. This would expand screening strategies to home-, mail-, or Internet-based screening, and encourage uptake of screening among younger persons at increased risk.

Relevance for Priority Populations

Expanding the range of specimen types for gonorrhea and chlamydia screening has the potential to increase identification of infected persons, particularly among priority populations. For example, the ability to test rectal and pharyngeal specimens may increase detection among MSM. Currently, NAATs are not FDA-cleared for use on rectal or pharyngeal sites in testing for gonorrhea and chlamydia. However, NAATs have improved sensitivity for detecting gonococcal infection at extragenital sites compared with culture in MSM, possibly because of lower bacterial loads at the pharynx and rectum.[61,62] Similar findings have been reported for chlamydia testing.[61] The prevalence of gonococcal and chlamydial infections varied by anatomical site in a study of MSM, which reported 53 percent of chlamydial and 64 percent of gonococcal infections occurring at rectal and pharyngeal sites, respectively.[63] In addition, 85 percent of rectal infections were asymptomatic and would only have been detected with routine screening. In another study of asymptomatic MSM, 84 percent of chlamydial and gonococcal infections were missed by testing for urethral infections only versus 9.8 percent of infections missed by screening only at the rectum and the pharynx.[60]

Future Research

Research is lacking on the effectiveness of screening for gonorrhea in all population groups and for chlamydia in men, pregnant women, and women without risk factors. Studies evaluating the effectiveness of different screening strategies for identifying persons at increased risk for infection, cotesting for concurrent STIs, and different screening intervals are needed to inform practice guidelines. For example, while no studies addressing repeat testing during pregnancy met inclusion criteria, an observational study conducted in the United States suggested that chlamydia test results in the first trimester may not predict chlamydia status during the third trimester.[56] Although studies of repeat testing have been conducted in some high-risk populations,[57] more research is warranted to further evaluate the value of repeat testing during pregnancy to reduce potential complications, such as preterm delivery and premature rupture of membranes.[58]

No studies provided data about potential adverse effects of screening other than those related to test performance for any of the asymptomatic population groups. An observational study of symptomatic and asymptomatic men and women who submitted self-collected specimens (from home) for chlamydia testing reported decreased anxiety after testing, although anxiety for women declined only after receiving negative results.[55] Waiting for test results generated anxiety and testing positive was associated with shock and distress for some participants, but many were glad that they had been tested. Additional studies on the harms of screening are needed.

Conclusions

Only one new trial of the effectiveness of screening for chlamydia in women,[26] one study of a risk prediction instrument,[29] and 10 studies of the diagnostic accuracy of screening tests met inclusion criteria. No studies addressed the effectiveness of screening for gonorrhea in all population groups and for chlamydia in men, pregnant women, and women without risk factors, or the effectiveness of different screening strategies. Aside from false-positive and false-negative findings, no studies provided data about other potential adverse effects of screening for any of the population groups. The findings of the POPI trial suggest benefits of screening for chlamydia for PID prevention, although results were not statistically significant. Screening with NAATs is accurate for diagnosing gonorrhea and chlamydia in asymptomatic persons regardless of specimen, anatomical site, or test. Further research is needed to understand the impact of screening for chlamydia and gonorrhea on clinical outcomes, effective screening strategies, and harms of screening.

REFERENCES

1.   U.S. Preventive Services Task Force. Screening for Gonorrhea: Recommendation Statement. Rockville, MD: Agency for Healthcare Research and Quality; 2005.
2.   U.S. Preventive Services Task Force. Screening for chlamydial infection: U.S. Preventive Services Task Force recommendation statement. *Ann Intern Med.* 2007;147(2):128-34.
3.   Nelson HD, Helfand M. Screening for chlamydial infection. *Am J Prev Med.* 2001;20(3 Suppl):95-107.
4.   Glass N, Nelson HD, Villemyer K. Screening for Gonorrhea: Update of the Evidence for the U.S. Preventive Services Task Force. Rockville, MD: Agency for Healthcare Research and Quality; 2005.
5.   Meyers DS, Halvorson H, Luckhaupt S; U.S. Preventive Services Task Force. Screening for chlamydial infection: an evidence update for the U.S. Preventive Services Task Force. *Ann Intern Med.* 2007;147(2):135-42.
6.   Merz AJ, So M. Interactions of pathogenic *Neisseriae* with epithelial cell membranes. *Annu Rev Cell Dev Biol.* 2000;16:423-57.
7.   Edwards JL, Apicella MA. The molecular mechanisms used by *Neisseria gonorrhoeae* to initiate infection differ between men and women. *Clin Microbiol Rev.* 2004;17(4):965-81.
8.   Centers for Disease Control and Prevention. 2012 Sexually Transmitted Disease Surveillance. Atlanta: Centers for Disease Control and Prevention; 2014. Accessed at http://www.cdc.gov/std/stats12/default.htm on 3 September 2014.
9.   Stephens RS. The cellular paradigm of chlamydial pathogenesis. *Trends Microbiol.* 2003;11(1):44-51.
10.   Centers for Disease Control and Prevention. Recommendations for the laboratory-based detection of *Chlamydia trachomatis* and *Neisseria gonorrhoeae*--2014. *MMWR Recomm Rep.* 2014;63(RR-02):1-19.
11.   Brocklehurst P. Antibiotics for gonorrhoea in pregnancy. *Cochrane Database Syst Rev.* 2002;(2):CD000098.
12.   Workowski KA, Levine WC; Centers for Disease Control and Prevention. Sexually transmitted disease treatment guidelines--2002. *MMWR Recomm Rep.* 2002;51(RR-06):1-78.
13.   Workowski KA, Berman S; Centers for Disease Control and Prevention. Sexually transmitted diseases treatment guidelines, 2010. *MMWR Recomm Rep.* 2010;59(RR-12):1-113.
14.   Workowski KA, Berman SM; Centers for Disease Control and Prevention. Sexually transmitted diseases treatment guidelines, 2006. *MMWR Recomm Rep.* 2006;55(RR-11):1-94.
15.   Centers for Disease Control and Prevention. CDC Grand Rounds: chlamydia prevention: challenges and strategies for reducing disease burden and sequelae. *MMWR Morb Mortal Wkly Rep.* 2011;60(12):370-3.
16.   Arya R, Mannion PT, Woodcock K, Haddad NG. Incidence of genital *Chlamydia trachomatis* infection in the male partners attending an infertility clinic. *J Obstet Gynaecol.* 2005;25(4):364-6.

17. Røttingen JA, Cameron WD, Garnett GP. A systematic review of the epidemiologic interactions between classic sexually transmitted diseases and HIV: how much really is known? *Sex Transm Dis*. 2001;28(10):579-97.

18. Baeten JM, Overbaugh J. Measuring the infectiousness of persons with HIV-1: opportunities for preventing sexual HIV-1 transmission. *Curr HIV Res*. 2003;1(1):69-86.

19. Centers for Disease Control and Prevention. Update to CDC's sexually transmitted diseases treatment guidelines, 2010: oral cephalosporins no longer a recommended treatment for gonococcal infections. *MMWR Morb Mortal Wkly Rep*. 2012;61(31):590-4.

20. Tao G, Irwin KL. Receipt of HIV and STD testing services during routine general medical or gynecological examinations: variations by patient sexual risk behaviors. *Sex Transm Dis*. 2008;35(2):167-71.

21. Centers for Disease Control and Prevention. Chlamydia screening among sexually active young female enrollees of health plans--United States, 2000-2007. *MMWR Morb Mortal Wkly Rep*. 2009;58(14):362-5.

22. Blatt AJ, Lieberman JM, Hoover DR, Kaufman HW. Chlamydial and gonococcal testing during pregnancy in the United States. *Am J Obstet Gynecol*. 2012;207(1):55.e1-8.

23. Harris RP, Helfand M, Woolf SH, Lohr KN, Mulrow CD, Teutsch SM, et al. Current methods of the U.S. Preventive Services Task Force: a review of the process. *Am J Prev Med*. 2001;20(3 Suppl):21-35.

24. U.S. Preventive Services Task Force. Procedure Manual. Rockville, MD: U.S. Preventive Services Task Force; 2011. Accessed at http://www.uspreventiveservicestaskforce.org/uspstf08/methods/procmanual.htm on 3 September 2014.

25. Centers for Disease Control and Prevention. Recall of LCx® *Neisseria gonorrhoeae* assay and implicatons for laboratory testing for *N. gonorrhoeae* and *Chlamydia trachomatis*. *MMWR Morb Mortal Wkly Rep*. 2002;51(32):709.

26. Oakeshott P, Kerry S, Aghaizu A, Atherton H, Hay S, Taylor-Robinson D, et al. Randomised controlled trial of screening for *Chlamydia trachomatis* to prevent pelvic inflammatory disease: the POPI (Prevention of Pelvic Infection) trial. *BMJ*. 2010;340:c1642.

27. Scholes D, Stergachis A, Heidrich FE, Andrilla H, Holmes KK, Stamm WE. Prevention of pelvic inflammatory disease by screening for cervical chlamydial infection. *N Engl J Med*. 1996;334(21):1362-6.

28. Ostergaard L, Andersen B, Møller JK, Olesen F. Home sampling versus conventional swab sampling for screening of *Chlamydia trachomatis* in women: a cluster-randomized 1-year follow-up study. *Clin Infect Dis*. 2000;31(4):951-7.

29. Götz HM, Veldhuijzen IK, Habbema JD, Boeke AJ, Richardus JH, Steyerberg EW. Prediction of *Chlamydia trachomatis* infection: application of a scoring rule to other populations. *Sex Transm Dis*. 2006;33(6):374-80.

30. Miller WC, Hoffman IF, Owen-O'Dowd J, McPherson JT, Privette A, Schmitz JL, et al. Selective screening for chlamydial infection: which criteria to use? *Am J Prev Med*. 2000;18(2):115-22.

31. Chernesky MA, Martin DH, Hook EW, Willis D, Jordan J, Wang S, et al. Ability of new APTIMA CT and APTIMA GC assays to detect *Chlamydia trachomatis* and *Neisseria gonorrhoeae* in male urine and urethral swabs. *J Clin Microbiol*. 2005;43(1):127-31.

32. Taylor SN, Liesenfeld O, Lillis RA, Body BA, Nye M, Williams J, et al. Evaluation of the Roche cobas® CT/NG test for detection of *Chlamydia trachomatis* and *Neisseria gonorrhoeae* in male urine. *Sex Transm Dis*. 2012;39(7):543-9.

33. Van Der Pol B, Liesenfeld O, Williams JA, Taylor SN, Lillis RA, Body BA, et al. Performance of the cobas CT/NG test compared to the APTIMA AC2 and Viper CTQ/GCQ assays for detection of *Chlamydia trachomatis* and *Neisseria gonorrhoeae*. *J Clin Microbiol*. 2012;50(7):2244-9.

34. Van Der Pol B, Taylor SN, Lebar W, Davis T, Fuller D, Mena L, et al. Clinical evaluation of the BD ProbeTec[TM] *Neisseria gonorrhoeae* Qx amplified DNA assay on the BD Viper[TM] system with XTR[TM] technology. *Sex Transm Dis*. 2012;39(2):147-53.

35. Stewart CM, Schoeman SA, Booth RA, Smith SD, Wilcox MH, Wilson JD. Assessment of self taken swabs versus clinician taken swab cultures for diagnosing gonorrhoea in women: single centre, diagnostic accuracy study. *BMJ*. 2012;345:e8107.

36. Gaydos CA, Van Der Pol B, Jett-Goheen M, Barnes M, Quinn N, Clark C, et al. Performance of the Cepheid CT/NG Xpert rapid PCR test for detection of *Chlamydia trachomatis* and *Neisseria gonorrhoeae*. *J Clin Microbiol*. 2013;51(6):1666-72.

37. Schachter J, McCormack WM, Chernesky MA, Martin DH, Van Der Pol B, Rice PA, et al. Vaginal swabs are appropriate specimens for diagnosis of genital tract infection with *Chlamydia trachomatis*. *J Clin Microbiol*. 2003;41(8):3784-9.

38. Shrier LA, Dean D, Klein E, Harter K, Rice PA. Limitations of screening tests for the detection of *Chlamydia trachomatis* in asymptomatic adolescent and young adult women. *Am J Obstet Gynecol*. 2004;190(3):654-62.

39. Taylor SN, Van Der Pol B, Lillis R, Hook EW 3rd, Lebar W, Davis T, et al. Clinical evaluation of the BD ProbeTec[TM] *Chlamydia trachomatis* Qx amplified DNA assay on the BD Viper[TM] system with XTR[TM] technology. *Sex Transm Dis*. 2011;38(7):603-9.

40. Schoeman SA, Stewart CM, Booth RA, Smith SD, Wilcox MH, Wilson JD. Assessment of best single sample for finding chlamydia in women with and without symptoms: a diagnostic test study. *BMJ*. 2012;345:e8013.

41. Pimenta JM, Catchpole M, Rogers PA, Hopwood J, Randall S, Mallinson H, et al. Opportunistic screening for genital chlamydial infection, II: prevalence among healthcare attenders, outcome, and evaluation of positive cases. *Sex Transm Infect*. 2003;79(1):22-7.

42. Burstein G, Jacobs A, Kissin D, Workowski K. Changes in the 2010 STD Treatment Guidelines: What Adolescent Health Care Providers Should Know. Washington, DC: American Congress of Obstetricians and Gynecologists; 2011. Accessed at http://www.acog.org/About-ACOG/ACOG-Departments/Adolescent-Health-Care/Changes-in-the-2010-STD-Treatment-Guidelines--What-Adolescent-Health-Care-Providers-Should-Know on 3 September 2014.

43. Moyer CS. STDs increasing among young women; more prevention urged. *American Medical News*. December 7, 2009. Accessed at http://www.amednews.com/article/20091207/profession/312079972/6/ on 3 September 2014.

44. Burstein G, Workowski K. What's new with 2010 STD treatment guidelines from the CDC? *AAP News*. 2011;32:7.

45. American Academy of Family Physicians. Clinical Preventive Services Recommendation: Chlamydia. Leawood, KS: American Academy of Family Physicians;

2007. Accessed at http://www.aafp.org/patient-care/clinical-recommendations/all/chlamydia.html on 3 September 2014.

46.   American College of Physicians. Clinical Practice Guidelines. Philadelphia: American College of Physicians; 2014. Accessed at http://www.acponline.org/clinical_information/guidelines/guidelines/ on 8 September 2014.

47.   Andersen B, van Valkengoed I, Sokolowski I, Møller JK, Østergaard L, Olesen F. Impact of intensified testing for urogenital *Chlamydia trachomatis* infections: a randomised study with 9-year follow-up. *Sex Transm Infect*. 2011;87(2):156-61.

48.   Low N, Egger M, Sterne JA, Harbord RM, Ibrahim F, Lindblom B, et al. Incidence of severe reproductive tract complications associated with diagnosed genital chlamydial infection: the Uppsala Women's Cohort Study. *Sex Transm Infect*. 2006;82(3):212-8.

49.   van den Broek IV, van Bergen JE, Brouwers EE, Fennema JS, Götz HM, Hoebe CJ, et al. Effectiveness of yearly, register based screening for chlamydia in the Netherlands: controlled trial with randomised stepped wedge implementation. *BMJ*. 2012;345:e4316.

50.   Scholes D, Satterwhite CL, Yu O, Fine D, Weinstock H, Berman S. Long-term trends in *Chlamydia trachomatis* infections and related outcomes in a U.S. managed care population. *Sex Transm Dis*. 2012;39(2):81-8.

51.   Gaydos CA, Barnes M, Jett-Goheen M, Quinn N, Whittle P, Hogan T, et al. Characteristics and predictors of women who obtain rescreening for sexually transmitted infections using the www.iwantthekit.org screening programme. *Int J STD AIDS*. 2013;24(9):736-44.

52.   Gottlieb SL, Stoner BP, Zaidi AA, Buckel C, Tran M, Leichliter JS, et al. A prospective study of the psychosocial impact of a positive *Chlamydia trachomatis* laboratory test. *Sex Transm Dis*. 2011;38(11):1004-11.

53.   Kangas I, Andersen B, Olesen F, Møller JK, Østergaard L. Psychosocial impact of *Chlamydia trachomatis* testing in general practice. *Br J Gen Pract*. 2006;56(529):587-93.

54.   Campbell R, Mills N, Sanford E, Graham A, Low N, Peters TJ; Chlamydia Screening Studies (ClaSS) Group. Does population screening for *Chlamydia trachomatis* raise anxiety among those tested? Findings from a population based chlamydia screening study. *BMC Public Health*. 2006;6:106.

55.   Low N, McCarthy A, Macleod J, Salisbury C, Campbell R, Roberts TE, et al. Epidemiological, social, diagnostic and economic evaluation of population screening for genital chlamydial infection. *Health Technol Assess*. 2007;11(8):iii-iv, ix-xii, 1-165.

56.   Hood EE, Nerhood RC. The utility of screening for chlamydia at 34-36 weeks gestation. *W V Med J*. 2010;106(6):10-1.

57.   Miller JM, Maupin RT, Nsuami M. Initial and repeat testing for chlamydia during pregnancy. *J Matern Fetal Neonatal Med*. 2005;18(4):231-5.

58.   Blas MM, Canchihuaman FA, Alva IE, Hawes SE. Pregnancy outcomes in women infected with *Chlamydia trachomatis*: a population-based cohort study in Washington State. *Sex Transm Infect*. 2007;83(4):314-8.

59.   Alexander S, Ison C, Parry J, Llewellyn C, Wayal S, Richardson D, et al. Self-taken pharyngeal and rectal swabs are appropriate for the detection of *Chlamydia trachomatis* and *Neisseria gonorrhoeae* in asymptomatic men who have sex with men. *Sex Transm Infect*. 2008;84(6):488-92.

60.   Marcus JL, Bernstein KT, Kohn RP, Liska S, Philip SS. Infections missed by urethral-only screening for chlamydia or gonorrhea detection among men who have sex with men. *Sex Transm Dis*. 2011;38(10):922-4.

61.   Schachter J, Moncada J, Liska S, Shayevich C, Klausner JD. Nucleic acid amplification tests in the diagnosis of chlamydial and gonococcal infections of the oropharynx and rectum in men who have sex with men. *Sex Transm Dis*. 2008;35(7):637-42.

62.   Bissessor M, Tabrizi SN, Fairley CK, Danielewski J, Whitton B, Bird S. Differing *Neisseria gonorrhoeae* bacterial loads in the pharynx and rectum in men who have sex with men: implications for gonococcal detection, transmission, and control. *J Clin Microbiol*. 2011;49(12):4304-6.

63.   Kent CK, Chaw JK, Wong W, Liska S, Gibson S, Hubbard G, et al. Prevalence of rectal, urethral, and pharyngeal chlamydia and gonorrhea detected in 2 clinical settings among men who have sex with men: San Francisco, California, 2003. *Clin Infect Dis*. 2005;41(1):67-74.

64.   Public Health Agency of Canada. Canadian Guidelines on Sexually Transmitted Infections. Ottawa, Ontario, Canada: Public Health Agency of Canada; 2010. Accessed at http://www.phac-aspc.gc.ca/std-mts/sti-its/ on 8 September 2014.

Figure 1. Analytic Framework: Screening in Men and Nonpregnant Women, Including Adolescents

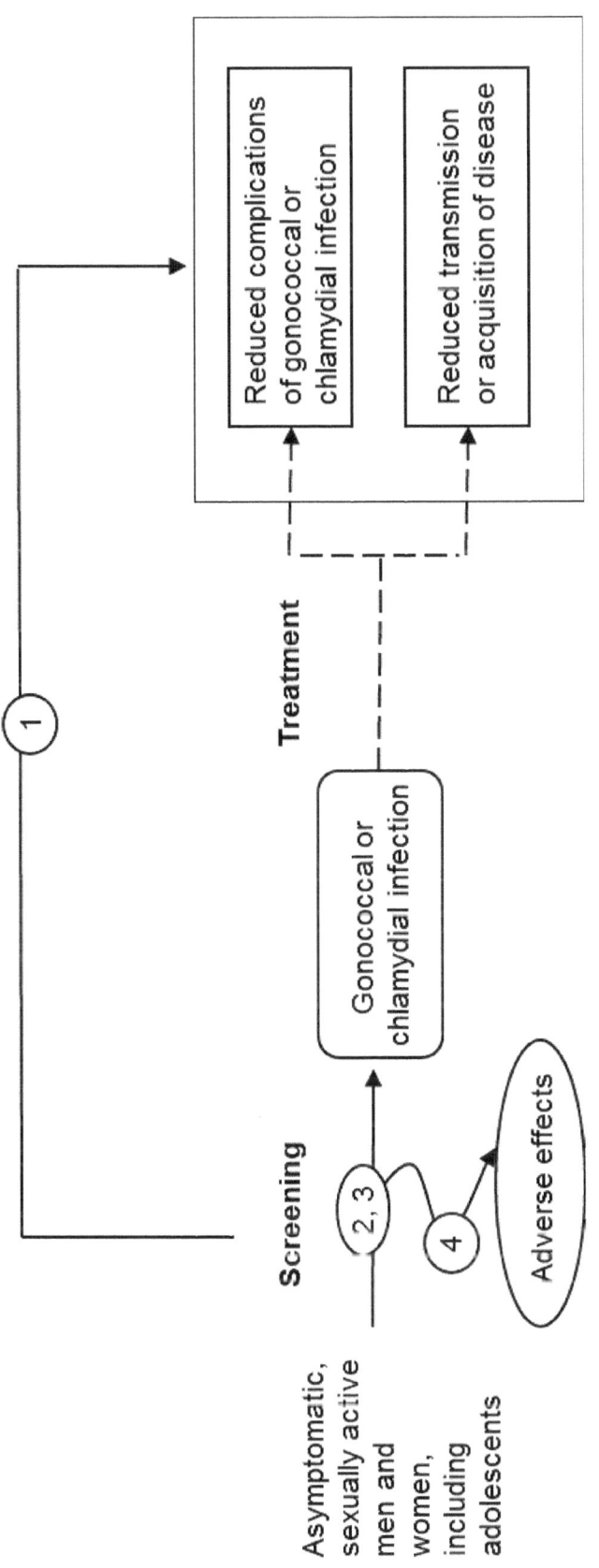

Key Questions

1. How effective is screening for gonorrhea and chlamydia in reducing complications of infection and transmission or acquisition of disease in asymptomatic, sexually active men and nonpregnant women, including adolescents?

2. How effective are different screening strategies in identifying persons with gonorrhea and chlamydia?

3. How accurate are screening tests for detecting gonorrhea and chlamydia?

4. What are the harms of screening for gonorrhea and chlamydia?

Figure 2. Analytic Framework: Screening in Pregnant Women

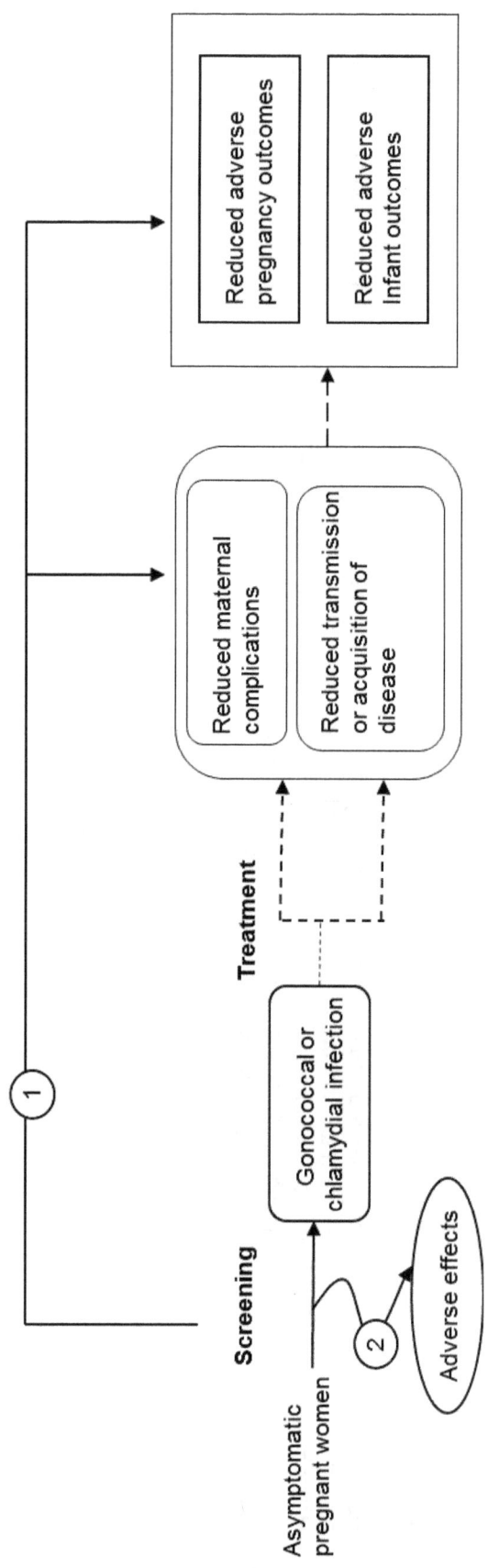

Key Questions

1. How effective is screening for gonorrhea and chlamydia in reducing maternal complications, adverse pregnancy and infant outcomes, and transmission or acquisition of disease in asymptomatic pregnant women?

2. What are the harms of screening for gonorrhea and chlamydia in asymptomatic pregnant women?

Figure 3. Diagnostic Accuracy of Nucleic Acid Amplification Tests for Screening for Gonorrhea in Men and Women

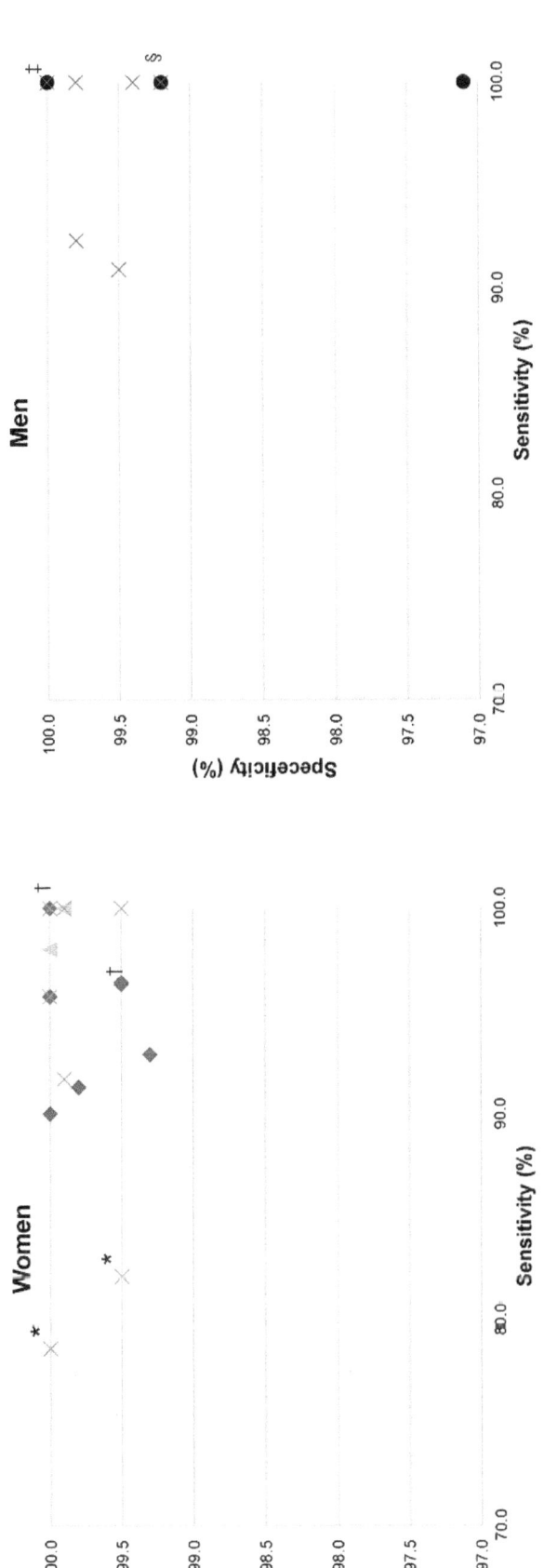

◆ Endocervix ▪ Clinician-Collected Vaginal ▲ Self Collected Vaginal × Urine ● Urethra

* The study reporting lower sensitivities for urine specimens in women (78.6% and 82.1%) used larger than recommended urine volumes,[34] differing from the other studies.

† Two studies produced identical data points for tests of the endocervix.

‡ Three data points for the urethra and three data points for urine.

§ Two data points for urethral samples.

Figure 4. Diagnostic Accuracy of Nucleic Acid Amplification Tests for Screening for Chlamydia in Women

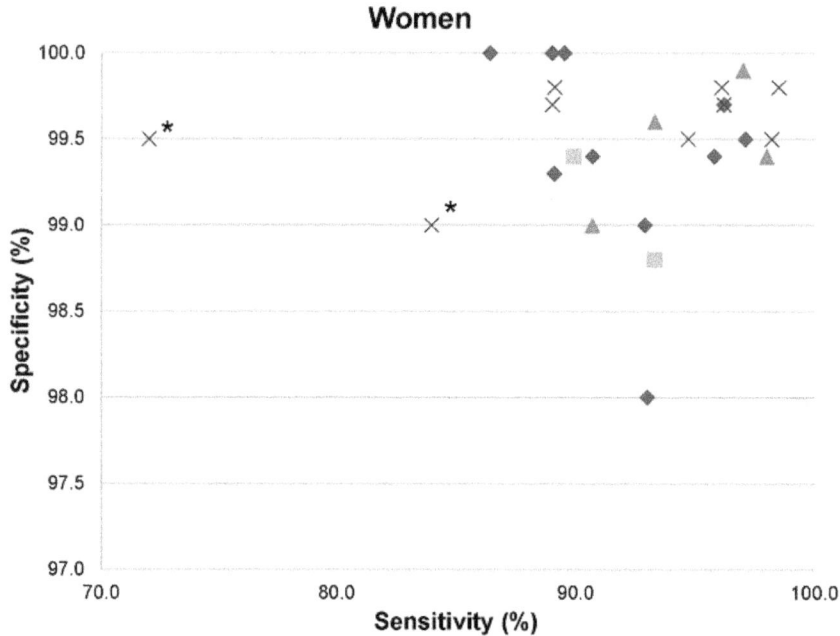

◆ Endocervix ▦ Clinician-Collected Vaginal ▲ Self Collected Vaginal ✕ Urine

*The study reporting lower sensitivities for urine specimens in women (72.0% and 84.0%) experienced technical and specimen processing errors,[37] differing from the other studies.

Figure 5. Diagnostic Accuracy of Nucleic Acid Amplification Tests for Screening for Chlamydia in Men

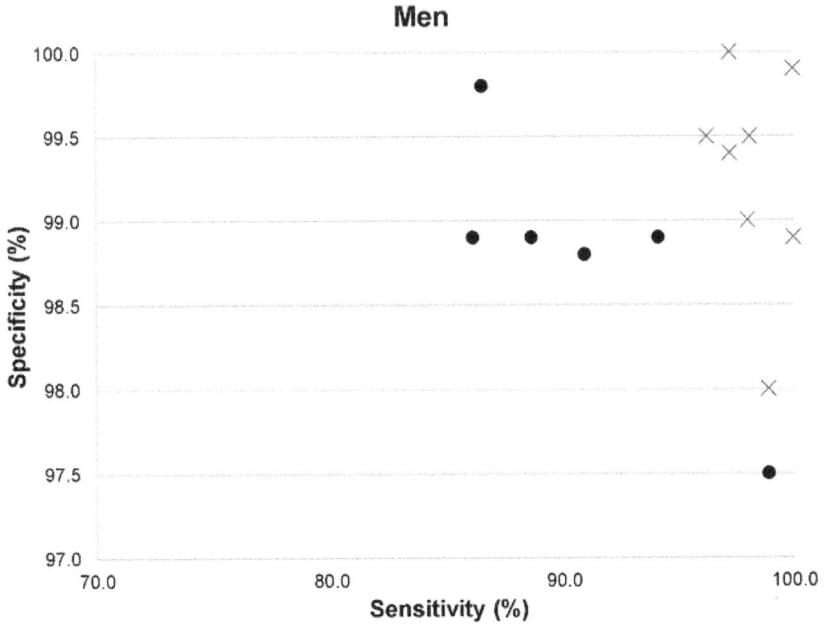

Table 1. Recommendations of Other Groups

Organization, year	Recommendations
Centers for Disease Control and Prevention (CDC), 2010[12]	The CDC recommendations are similar to those of the USPSTF for screening for gonorrhea in men and women. The CDC recommends annual screening for chlamydia in all sexually active women age ≤25 years and in older women with specific risk factors (e.g., a new or multiple sex partners) and screening for gonorrhea in sexually active women at increased risk for infection (e.g., those age <25 years). Because of high rates of reinfection, retesting for gonorrhea and chlamydia in infected persons is recommended 3 months after treatment. Routine screening for gonorrhea and chlamydia in the general population, including men, is not recommended. Clinical settings with a high prevalence of chlamydia should consider screening in sexually active young men. Also, adolescent and adult females age ≤35 years should be screened for gonorrhea and chlamydia at intake in juvenile detention or jail facilities. The CDC recommends screening annually for gonorrhea and chlamydia in men who have sex with men, based on exposure history, with more frequent screening recommended in highest-risk populations. High-risk pregnant women should be screened for gonorrhea and all pregnant women should be screened for chlamydia at their first prenatal visit. Pregnant women who continue to be at risk for these infections and those who test positive at their first prenatal visit should be retested in the third trimester.
American Congress of Obstetricians and Gynecologists (ACOG), 2010[42]	ACOG recommends annual screening for gonorrhea in high-risk females age <25 years. Annual screening for chlamydia is recommended in all sexually active females age ≤25 years. Adolescent and young adult males presenting to clinics associated with high chlamydia prevalence may be considered for screening.
American Medical Association, 2009[43]	Follow CDC recommendations.
American Academy of Pediatrics, 2011[44]	Follow CDC recommendations
American Academy of Family Physicians, 2007[45]	Follow USPSTF recommendations.
American College of Physicians, 2007[46]	Follow USPSTF recommendations.
Public Health Agency of Canada, 2010[64]	The Canadian guidelines recommend screening for gonorrhea and chlamydia in at-risk groups, including all sexually active males and females age <25 years, with repeat screening after 6 months in infected persons. Pregnant women should be screened for gonorrhea and chlamydia at the first prenatal visit and again during the third trimester for those who test positive or are high risk.

Table 2. Randomized, Controlled Trials of Screening for Chlamydia to Reduce Adverse Health Outcomes

Author, Year	Population, n	Interventions	Duration	Attrition	Independent testing*	Outcomes	Quality
Oakeshott et al, 2010[26] (see text)	2,529 sexually active women age ≤27 years recruited from universities and colleges in the United Kingdom.	Immediate screening vs. deferred screening after 1 year (control)	1 year	Screened: 5% Control: 7%	Screened: 23% Control: 22%	Incidence of PID in asymptomatic women (n=1,648): Screened: 0.6% (5/787) Control: 1.6% (14/861) RR, 0.39 (95% CI, 0.14 to 1.08) Incidence of PID in all women: Screened: 1.3% (15/1191) Control: 1.9% (23/1186) RR, 0.65 (95% CI, 0.34 to 1.22)	Good
Prior reports							
Ostergaard et al, 2000[28]	1,700 female students recruited from high schools in one county in Denmark.	Home screening vs. usual care opportunistic screening in a clinic (control)	1 year	Screened: 49% Control: 42%	Screened: 29% Control: 36%	Incidence of new chlamydial infections in all females: Screened: 2.9% (13/443) Control: 6.6% (32/487) RR, 0.45 (95% CI, 0.24 to 0.84)[†] p=0.026 Incidence of PID in all females: Screened: 2.1% (9/443) Control: 4.2% (20/487) RR, 0.50 (95% CI, 0.23 to 1.08)[†] p=0.045	Poor[‡]
Scholes et al, 1996[27]	2,607 women ages 18 to 34 years recruited from a health maintenance organization in the United States, selected by risk criteria.	Clinic screening vs. usual care (control)	1 year	24% of participants did not return final questionnaire	Not reported	Incidence of PID in all women: Screened: 8 per 10,000 women-years (9 cases) Control: 18 per 10,000 women-years (33 cases) RR, 0.44 (95% CI, 0.20 to 0.90)	Good[‡]

*Only includes participants with followup who were independently tested outside of study protocol.
†Calculated.
‡As rated by prior review authors

Abbreviations: CI = confidence interval; PID = pelvic inflammatory disease; RR = relative risk.

Table 3. Included Studies of Nucleic Acid Amplification Tests for Screening for Gonorrhea and Chlamydia At Various Anatomical Sites

Test	Anatomical site						
	Endocervix	Clinician-collected vagina	Self-collected vagina	Male urethra	Urine	Rectum	Pharynx
Gonorrhea							
GenProbe APTIMA COMBO 2	Van Der Pol et al, 2012[33] Van Der Pol et al, 2012[34] Stewart et al, 2012[35]	No studies	Stewart et al, 2012[46]	Taylor et al, 2012[32] Van Der Pol et al, 2012[34]	Taylor et al, 2012[32] Van Der Pol et al, 2012[33] Van Der Pol et al, 2012[34]	Not FDA approved site	Not FDA approved site
GenProbe APTIMA GC	No studies found	No studies	No studies	Chernesky et al, 2005[31]	Chernesky et al,2005[31]	Not FDA approved site	Not FDA approved site
BD ProbeTec ET	Van Der Pol et al, 2012[34]	No studies	No studies	Van Der Pol et al, 2012[34]	Van Der Pol et al, 2012[34]	Not FDA approved site	Not FDA approved site
BD ProbeTec CT/GC Q[x] Amplified DNA Assay	Van Der Pol et al, 2012[33] Van Der Pol et al, 2012[34] Stewart et al, 2012[35]	No studies	No studies	Taylor et al, 2012[32] Van Der Pol et al, 2012[34]	Taylor et al, 2012[32] Van Der Pol et al, 2012[33] Van Der Pol et al, 2012[34]	Not FDA approved site	Not FDA approved site
Roche COBAS CT/NG test (c4800)	Van Der Pol et al, 2012[33] Van Der Pol et al, 2012[34] Stewart et al, 2012[35]	No studies	No studies	No studies	Taylor et al, 2012[32] Van Der Pol et al, 2012[33]	Not FDA approved site	Not FDA approved site
Cepheid GeneXpert CT/NG	Gaydos et al, 2013[36]	Not FDA approved site	Gaydos et al, 2013[36]	Not FDA approved site	Gaydos et al, 2013[36]	Not FDA approved site	Not FDA approved site
Chlamydia							
Roche COBAS AMPLICOR CT/NG Test	Schachter et al, 2003[37] Shrier et al, 2004[38]	Schachter et al, 2003[37] Shrier et al, 2004[38]	Schachter et al, 2003[37] Shrier et al, 2004[38]	No studies	Schachter et al, 2003[37] Shrier et al, 2004[38]	Not FDA approved site	Not FDA approved site
GenProbe APTIMA COMBO 2	Taylor et al, 2011[39] Van Der Pol et al, 2012[33] Schoeman et al, 2012[40]	No studies	Schoeman et al, 2012[40]	Taylor et al, 2012[32] Taylor et al, 2011[39]	Taylor et al, 2012[32] Taylor et al, 2011[39] Van Der Pol et al, 2012[33]	Not FDA approved site	Not FDA approved site
GenProbe APTIMA CT	Schachter et al, 2003[40]	Schachter et al, 2003[40]	Schachter et al, 2003[40]	Chernesky et al, 2005[31]	Schachter et al, 2003[37] Chernesky et al, 2005[31]	Not FDA approved site	Not FDA approved site
BD ProbeTec ET	Taylor et al, 2011[39]	No studies	No studies	Taylor et al, 2011[39]	Taylor et al, 2011[39]	Not FDA approved site	Not FDA approved site
BD ProbeTec CT/GC Q[x] Amplified DNA Assay	Taylor et al, 2011[39] Van Der Pol et al, 2012[33]	No studies	No studies	Taylor et al, 2012[32]; Taylor et al, 2011[39]	Taylor et al, 2012[32] Taylor et al, 2011[39] Van Der Pol et al, 2012[33]	Not FDA approved site	Not FDA approved site
Roche COBAS CT/NG test (c4800)	Van Der Pol et al, 2012[33]	No studies	No studies	No studies	Taylor et al, 2012[32] Van Der Pol et al, 2012[33]	Not FDA approved site	Not FDA approved site

Table 3. Included Studies of Nucleic Acid Amplification Tests for Screening for Gonorrhea and Chlamydia At Various Anatomical Sites

Cepheid GeneXpert CT/NG	Gaydos et al, 2015[36]	Not FDA approved site	Gaydos et al, 2013[36]	Not FDA approved site	Gaydos et al, 2013[36]	Not FDA approved site

Abbreviations: BD = Becton Dickinson; CT = *Chlamydia trachomatis*; ET = FDA = U.S. Food and Drug Administration; GC = gonorrhea/chlamydia; NG = *Neisseria gonorrhea*.

Table 4. Diagnostic Accuracy of Nucleic Acid Amplification Tests for Screening for Gonorrhea in Women

Test	Definition of a positive screening test	Reference standard	Prevalence (%)	TP (n)	FP (n)	FN (n)	TN (n)	Sens (%)	Spec (%)	PPV (%)	NPV (%)	PLR	NLR
Endocervix													
TMA[33]	Positive result from ≥2 NAATs with different target regions in endocervical swab and/or FCU; each NAAT was evaluated based on results of other 2 NAATs	TMA SDA	1.5	23	0	0	2266	100.0	100.0	100.0*	100.0*	Unable to calculate	0.00*
TMA[34]	≥1 positive result from each reference NAAT; for assay comparison, positive result required from each of other 2 assays	TMA SDA	6.5	27	2	1	418	96.4	99.5	93.1*	99.8*	202.5*	0.04*
PCR[33]	Positive result from ≥2 NAATs with different target regions in endocervical swab and/or FCU; each NAAT was evaluated based on results of other 2 NAATs	TMA SDA	1.5	22	0	1	2246	95.7	100.0	100.0*†	100.0*	Unable to calculate	0.04*
SDA[33]	Positive result from ≥2 NAATs with different target regions in endocervical swab and/or FCU; each NAAT was evaluated based on results of other 2 NAATs	TMA SDA	1.5	21	4	2	2241	91.3	99.8	84.0*	99.9*	512.5*	0.09*
SDA[34]	≥1 positive result from each reference NAAT; for assay comparison, positive result from each of other 2 assays	TMA SDA	6.5	26	2	1	421	96.3	99.5	92.9*	99.8*	203.7*	0.04*
SDA[34]	≥1 positive result from each reference NAAT; for assay comparison, positive result from each of other 2 assays	TMA SDA	6.5	26	3	2	407	92.9	99.3	89.7*	99.5*	126.9*	0.07*
TMA[35]	Positive culture with biochemical confirmation or positive result from 1 NAAT confirmed by second NAAT	Culture TMA	2.5	36	0	4	2194	90.0	100.0	100.0*	98.8*	Unable to calculate	0.10*
PCR[36]	≥1 positive result from each reference NAAT	TMA SDA	1.1	12	0	0	1116	100.0	100.0	100.0	100.0	Unable to calculate	0.00*
Self-collected vaginal													
TMA[35]	Positive culture with biochemical confirmation or positive result from 1 NAAT confirmed by second NAAT	Culture TMA	2.5	39	0	1	2194	98.0	100.0*	100.0*	100.0*	Unable to calculate	0.03*
PCR[36]	≥1 positive result from each reference NAAT	TMA SDA	1.1	12	1	0	1119	100.0	99.9	92.3	100	1120.0*	0.00*
First-catch urine													
TMA[34]	≥1 positive result from each reference NAAT; for assay comparison, positive result required from each of other 2 assays	TMA SDA	6.5	22	0	6	422	78.6	100.0	100.0*	98.6*	Unable to calculate	0.21*
TMA[33]	Positive result from ≥2 NAATs with different target regions in endocervical swab and/or FCU; each NAAT was evaluated based on results of other 2 NAATs	TMA SDA	1.5	22	1	1	2268	95.7	100.0	95.7*	100.0*	2170.4*	0.04*

Table 4. Diagnostic Accuracy of Nucleic Acid Amplification Tests for Screening for Gonorrhea in Women

Test	Definition of a positive screening test	Reference standard	Prevalence (%)	TP (n)	FP (n)	FN (n)	TN (n)	Sens (%)	Spec (%)	PPV (%)	NPV (%)	PLR	NLR
PCR[33]	Positive result from ≥2 NAATs with different target regions in endocervical swab and/or FCU; each NAAT was evaluated based on results of other 2 NAATs	TMA SDA	1.5	23	1	0	2255	100.0	100.0	95.8*	100.0*	2256.0*	0.00*
SDA[33]	Positive result from ≥2 NAATs with different target regions in endocervical swab and/or FCU; each NAAT was evaluated based on results of other 2 NAATs	TMA SDA	1.5	23	3	0	2246	100.0	99.9	88.5*	100.0*	749.7*	0.00*
SDA[34]	≥1 positive result from each reference NAAT; for assay comparison, positive result required from each of other 2 assays	TMA SDA	6.5	27	2	0	421	100.0	99.5	93.1*	100.0*	211.5*	0.00*
SDA[34]	≥1 positive result from each reference NAAT; for assay comparison, positive result required from each of other 2 assays	TMA SDA	6.5	23	2	5	414	82.1	99.5	92.0*	98.8*	170.9*	0.18*
PCR[36]	≥1 positive result from each reference NAAT	TMA SDA	1.1	11	1	1	1123	91.7	99.9	91.7	99.9	1030.3*	0.08*

*Calculated.
†Estimated PPV, 93.8% to 99.9% (based on hypothetical prevalence range of 1% to 50%).

Abbreviations: FCU = first-catch urine; FN = false negative; FP = false positive; n = number; NAAT = nucleic acid amplification test; NG = *Neisseria gonorrhea*; NLR = negative likelihood ratio; NPV = negative predictive value; PCR = polymerase chain reaction; PLR = positive likelihood ratio; PPV = positive predictive value; SDA = strand displacement assay; Sens = sensitivity; Spec = specificity; TMA = transcription-mediated assay; TN = true negative; TP = true positive.

Table 5. Diagnostic Accuracy of Nucleic Acid Amplification Tests for Screening for Gonorrhea in Men

Test	Definition of a positive screening test	Reference standard	Prevalence (%)	TP (n)	FP (n)	FN (n)	TN (n)	Sens (%)	Spec (%)	PPV (%)	NPV (%)	PLR	NLR
Urethra													
TMA[31]	Both urethral swab and FCU positive on ≥1 of 2 NAATs; or positive on both tests for ≥1 specimen type	TMA SDA	13.8	110	21	0	710	100.0	97.1	84.0*	100.0*	34.8*	0.00*
TMA[32]	Positive result from ≥2 NAATs with different target regions in urethral swab and/or FCU	TMA SDA	9.2	7	0	0	465	100.0	100.0	100.0*	100.0*	Unable to calculate	0.00*
TMA[34]	≥1 positive result from each reference NAAT; for assay comparison, positive result required from each of other 2 assays	TMA SDA	14.5	11	4	0	469	100.0	99.2	73.3*	100.0*	118.3*	0.00*
SDA[32]	Positive result from ≥2 NAATs with different target regions in urethral swab and/or FCU	TMA SDA	9.2	7	0	0	465	100.0	100.0	100.0*	100.0*	Unable to calculate	0.00*
SDA[34]	≥1 positive result from each reference NAAT; for assay comparison, positive result required from each of other 2 assays	TMA SDA	14.5	12	4	0	492	100.0	99.2	75.0*	100.0*	124.0*	0.00*
SDA[34]	≥1 positive result from each reference NAAT; for assay comparison, positive result required from each of other 2 assays	TMA SDA	14.5	12	0	0	480	100.0	100.0	100.0*	100.0*	Unable to calculate	0.00*
First-catch urine													
TMA[31]	Both urethral swab and FCU positive on ≥1 of 2 NAATs; or positive on both tests for ≥1 specimen type	TMA SDA	13.8	100	4	10	730	90.9	99.5	96.2*	98.7*	166.8*	0.09*
TMA[34]	≥1 positive result from each reference NAAT; for assay comparison, positive result required from each of other 2 assays	TMA SDA	14.5	12	3	0	502	100.0	99.4	80.0*	100.0*	168.3*	0.00*
TMA[32]	Positive result from ≥2 NAATs with different target regions in urethral swab and/or FCU	TMA SDA	9.2	7	0	0	465	100.0	100.0	100.0*	100.0*	Unable to calculate	0.00*
PCR[32]	Positive result from ≥2 NAATs with different target regions in urethral swab and/or FCU	TMA SDA	9.2	7	0	0	465	100.0	100.0	100.0*	100.0*	Unable to calculate	0.00*
SDA[32]	Positive result from ≥2 NAATs with different target regions in urethral swab and/or FCU	TMA SDA	9.2	7	1	0	464	100.0	99.8	87.5*	100.0*	465.0*	0.00*
SDA[34]	≥1 positive result from each reference NAAT; for assay comparison, positive result required from each of other 2 assays	TMA SDA	14.5	12	4	0	501	100.0	99.2	75.0*	100.0*	126.3*	0.00*
SDA[34]	≥1 positive result from each reference NAAT; for assay comparison, positive result required from each of other 2 assays	TMA SDA	14.5	12	1	1	497	92.3	99.8	92.3*	99.8*	459.7*	0.08*
PCR[35]	≥1 positive result from each reference NAAT	TMA SDA	0.4	5	1	0	1126	100	99.9	83.3	100	1127.0*	0.00*

* Calculated.

Abbreviations: FCU = first-catch urine; FN = false negative; FP = false positive; n = number; NAAT = nucleic acid amplification test; NLR = negative likelihood ratio; NPV = negative predictive value; PCR = polymerase chain reaction; PLR = positive likelihood ratio; PPV = positive predictive value; SDA = strand displacement assay; Sens = sensitivity; Spec = specificity; TMA = transcription-mediated amplification; TN = true negative; TP = true positive.

Table 6. Diagnostic Accuracy of Nucleic Acid Amplification Tests for Screening for Gonorrhea and Chlamydia at Various Anatomical Sites

Test	Studies	Endocervix Sens (%)	Endocervix Spec (%)	Clinician-collected vagina Sens (%)	Clinician-collected vagina Spec (%)	Self-collected vagina Sens (%)	Self-collected vagina Spec (%)	Male urethra Sens (%)	Male urethra Spec (%)	Urine Sens (%)	Urine Spec (%)
Gonorrhea											
GenProbe APTIMA COMBO 2	Van Der Pol et al, 2012[33]	100.0	100.0							F: 95.7	F: 100.0
	Van Der Pol et al, 2012[34]	96.4	99.5					100.0	99.2	F: 78.6 M: 100.0	F: 100.0 M: 99.4
	Stewart et al, 2012[35]	90.0	100.0			98.0	100.0				
	Taylor et al, 2012[32]							100.0	100.0	M: 100.0	M: 100.0
GenProbe APTIMA GC	Chemesky et al, 2005[31]							100	97.1	M: 90.9	M: 99.5
BD ProbeTec ET	Van Der Pol et al, 2012[34]	92.9	99.3					100.0	100.0	F: 82.1 M: 92.3	F: 99.5 M: 99.8
BD ProbeTec CT/GC Q^X Amplified DNA Assay	Van Der Pol et al, 2012[33]	91.3	99.8							F: 100.0	F: 99.9
	Van Der Pol et al, 2012[34]	96.3	99.5					100.0	99.2	F: 100.0 M: 100.0	F: 99.5 M: 99.2
	Taylor et al, 2012[32]							100.0	100.0	M: 100.0	M: 99.8
Roche COBAS CT/NG Test (c4800)	Van Der Pol et al, 2012[33]	95.7	100.0							F: 100.0	F: 100.0
	Taylor et al, 2012[32]									M: 100.0	M: 100.0
Cepheid GeneXpert CT/NG	Gaydos et al, 2013[36]	100.0	100.0			100.0	99.9			F: 91.7 M: 100.0	F: 99.9 M: 99.9
Chlamydia											
Roche COBAS	Schachter et al, 2003[37]	90.7	99.4	93.3	98.8	90.7	99.0			F: 84.0	F: 99.9
	Shrier et al, 2004[38]	51.9	100.0	55.6	100.0	51.9	99.0			F: 44.4	F: 100.0
GenProbe APTIMA COMBO 2	Schoenan et al, 2012[40]	89.0	100.0			97.0	99.9				
	Taylor et al, 2012[32]	92.9	99.0					94.1	98.9	M: 98.0	M: 99.0
	Taylor et al, 2011[39]							90.9	98.8	F: 98.2 M: 97.2	F: 99.5 M: 100.0
GenProbe APTIMA CT	Van Der Pol et al, 2012[33]	97.1	99.5							F: 92.5	F: 99.8
	Schachter et al, 2003[37]	89.1	99.3	89.9	99.4	93.3	99.6			F: 72.0	F: 99.5
BD ProbeTec ET	Chernesky et al, 2005[31]							98.9	97.5	M: 98.9	M: 98.0
	Taylor et al, 2011[39]	86.4	100.0					86.1	98.9	F: 89.8 M: 97.2	F: 99.7 M:99.4
BD ProbeTec CT/GC Q^X Amplified DNA Assay	Taylor et al, 2012[32]	93.0	98.0					86.5	99.8	M: 96.2	M: 99.5
	Taylor et al, 2011[39]							88.6	98.9	F: 94.7 M: 100.0	F: 99.5 M: 98.9
	Van Der Pol et al, 2012[33]	96.2	99.7							F: 96.2	F: 99.7
	Taylor et al, 2012[32]									M: 98.1	M: 99.5
Roche COBAS CT/NG Test (c4800)	Van Der Pol et al, 2012[33]	89.5	100.0							F: 89.1	F: 99.8
Cepheid GeneXpert CT/NG	Gaydos et al, 2013[36]	95.8	99.4			98.0	99.4			F: 96.1 M: 100.0	F: 99.8 M: 99.9

Abbreviations: BC = Becton Dickinson; CT = *Chlamydia trachomatis*; F = female; GC = gonorrhea/chlamydia; M = male; NG = *Neisseria gonorrhea*; Sens = sensitivity; Spec = specificity.

Table 7. Diagnostic Accuracy of Nucleic Acid Amplification Tests for Screening for Chlamydia in Women

Test	Definition of a positive screening test	Reference standard	Prevalence (%)	TP (n)	FP (n)	FN (n)	TN (n)	Sens (%)	Spec (%)	PPV (%)	NPV (%)	PLR	NLR
Endocervix													
TMA[37]	Agreement between positive results with vaginal swab and cervical swab or FCU	Culture	9.6	106*	10	13*	1262*	89.1	99.3	91.4*	99.0*	113.3*	0.11*
TMA[39]	≥1 positive result from each reference NAAT; for assay comparison, positive result required from each of other 2 assays	TMA SDA	11.6	52	4	4	389	92.9	99.0	92.9*	99.0*	91.2*	0.07*
TMA[33]	Positive result from ≥2 NAATs with different target regions in endocervical swab and/or FCU; each NAAT was evaluated based on results of other 2 NAATs	TMA SDA	6.3	101	12	3	2173	97.1	99.5	89.4*	99.9*	176.8*	0.03*
TMA[40]	Positive result from 1 NAAT confirmed by second NAAT	TMA	10.3	163	0	20	2050	89.0	100.0	100.0	99.0	Unable to calculate	0.11*
PCR[33]	Positive result from ≥2 NAATs with different target regions in endocervical swab and/or FCU; each NAAT was evaluated based on results of other 2 NAATs	TMA SDA	6.3	94	1	11	2163	89.5	100.0	99.0*†	99.5*	1937.3*	0.10*
PCR[37]	Agreement between positive results with vaginal swab and cervical swab or FCU	Culture	9.6	68*	3	7*	503*	90.7	99.4	95.8*	98.6*	152.9*	0.09*
PCR[38]	1 positive culture or 2 positive nonculture tests, or 1 positive nonculture test confirmed by nested PCR	Culture PCR LCR	21.6	14	0	13	99	51.9	100.0	100.0	88.4	Unable to calculate	0.48*
SDA[33]	Positive result from ≥2 NAATs with different target regions in endocervical swab and/or FCU; each NAAT was evaluated based on results of other 2 NAATs	TMA SDA	6.3	102	7	4	2155	96.2	99.7	93.6*	99.8*	297.2*	0.04*
SDA[39]	≥1 positive result from each reference NAAT; for assay comparison, positive result required from each of other 2 assays	TMA SDA	11.6	53	8	4	385	93.0	98.0	86.9*	99.0*	45.7*	0.07*
SDA[39]	≥1 positive result from each reference NAAT; for assay comparison, positive result required from each of other 2 assays	TMA SDA	11.6	51	0	8	379	86.4	100.0	100.0*	97.9*	Unable to calculate	0.14*
PCR[36]	≥1 positive result from each reference NAAT	TMA SDA	4.3	46	6	2	1074	95.8	99.4	88.5	99.8	172.5*	0.04*

Table 7. Diagnostic Accuracy of Nucleic Acid Amplification Tests for Screening for Chlamydia in Women

Test	Definition of a positive screening test	Reference standard	Prevalence (%)	TP (n)	FP (n)	FN (n)	TN (n)	Sens (%)	Spec (%)	PPV (%)	NPV (%)	PLR	NLR
First-catch urine													
TMA[37]	Agreement between positive results with vaginal swab and cervical swab or FCU	Culture	9.6	86*	7	33*	1265*	72.0	99.5	92.5*	97.5*	131.3*	0.28*
TMA[33]	Positive result from ≥2 NAATs with different target regions in endocervical swab and/or FCU; each NAAT was evaluated based on results of other 2 NAATs	TMA SDA	6.3	98	5	8	2181	92.5	99.8	95.2*	99.6*	404.2*	0.08*
TMA[39]	≥1 positive result from each reference NAAT; for assay comparison, positive result required from each of other 2 assays	TMA SDA	11.6	55	2	1	392	98.2	99.5	96.5*	99.8*	193.5*	0.02*
PCR[33]	Positive result from ≥2 NAATs with different target regions in endocervical swab and/or FCU; each NAAT was evaluated based on results of other 2 NAATs	TMA SDA	6.3	98	4	12	2165	89.1	99.8	96.1*	99.5*	483.1*	0.11*
PCR[37]	Agreement between positive results with vaginal swab and cervical swab or FCU	Culture	9.6	63*	5	12*	501*	84.0	99.0	92.7*	97.7*	85.0*	0.16*
PCR[38]	1 positive culture or 2 positive nonculture tests, or 1 positive nonculture test confirmed by nested PCR	Culture PCR LCR	21.6	12	0	15	99	44.4	100.0	100.0	86.8	0.56*	Unable to calculate
SDA[33]	Positive result from ≥2 NAATs with different target regions in endocervical swab and/or FCU; each NAAT was evaluated based on results of other 2 NAATs	TMA SDA	6.3	101	6	4	2161	96.2	99.7	94.4*	99.8*	347.4*	0.04*
SDA[39]	≥1 positive result from each reference NAAT; for assay comparison, positive result required from each of other 2 assays	TMA SDA	11.6	54	2	3	391	94.7	99.5	96.4*	99.2*	186.2*	0.05*
SDA[39]	≥1 positive result from each reference NAAT; for assay comparison, positive result required from each of other 2 assays	TMA SDA	11.6	53	1	6	384	89.8	99.7	98.2*	98.5*	345.9*	0.10*
PCR[36]	≥1 positive result from each reference NAAT	TMA SDA	4.5	49	2	2	1083	96.1	99.8	96.1	99.8	521.2*	0.04*
Clinician-collected vaginal													
TMA[37]	Agreement between positive results with vaginal swab and cervical swab or FCU	Culture	9.6	107*	9	12*	1263*	89.9	99.4	92.2*	99.1*	127.1*	0.10*

Table 7. Diagnostic Accuracy of Nucleic Acid Amplification Tests for Screening for Chlamydia in Women

Test	Definition of a positive screening test	Reference standard	Prevalence (%)	TP (n)	FP (n)	FN (n)	TN (n)	Sens (%)	Spec (%)	PPV (%)	NPV (%)	PLR	NLR
PCR[37]	Agreement between positive results with vaginal swab and cervical swab or FCU	Culture	9.6	70*	6	5*	500*	93.3	98.8	92.1*	99.0*	78.7*	0.07**
PCR[38]	1 positive culture or 2 positive nonculture tests, or 1 positive nonculture test confirmed by nested PCR	Culture PCR LCR	21.6	15	0	12	99	55.6	100.0	100.0*	89.2*	Unable to calculate	0.44*
Self-collected vaginal													
TMA[37]	Agreement between positive results with vaginal swab and cervical swab or FCU	Culture	9.6	111*	6	8*	1266*	93.3	99.6	94.9	99.4	197.8*	0.07*
PCR[37]	Agreement between positive results with vaginal swab and cervical swab or FCU	Culture	9.6	68*	5	7*	501*	90.7	99.0	93.2	98.6*	91.8*	0.09*
PCR[38]	1 positive culture or 2 positive nonculture tests, or 1 positive nonculture test confirmed by nested PCR	Culture PCR LCR	21.6	14	1	13	98	51.9	99.0	93.3	83.3	51.3*	0.49*
TMA[40]	Positive result from 1 NAAT confirmed by second NAAT	TMA	10.3	178	1	5	2049	97.0	99.9	99.4*	99.8*	1994.0*	0.03*
PCR[36]	≥1 positive result from each reference NAAT	TMA SDA	4.3	48	7	1	1076	98.0	99.4	87.3	99.9	151.6*	0.02*

*Calculated.
†Estimated PPV, 77.3% to 99.7% (based on hypothetical prevalence range of 1% to 50%).

Abbreviations: FCU = first-catch urine; FN = false negative; FP = false positive; LCR = ligase chain reaction; n = number; NAAT = nucleic acid amplification test; NLR = negative likelihood ratio; NPV = negative predictive value; PCR = polymerase chain reaction; PLR = positive likelihood ratio; PPV = positive predictive value; SDA = strand displacement assay; Sens = sensitivity; Spec = specificity; TMA = transcription-mediated amplification; TN = true negative; TP = true positive.

Table 8. Diagnostic Accuracy of Nucleic Acid Amplification Tests for Screening for Chlamydia in Men

Test	Definition of a positive screening test	Reference standard	Prevalence (%)	TP (n)	FP (n)	FN (n)	TN (n)	Sens (%)	Spec (%)	PPV (%)	NPV (%)	PLR	NLR
Urethra													
TMA[31]	Positive result from ≥1 NAAT in both urethral swab and FCU; or 1 specimen positive on both NAATs	TMA SDA	17.9	94	16	1	634	98.9	97.5	85.5*	99.8*	40.2*	0.01*
TMA[32]	Positive result from ≥2 NAATs with different target regions in urethral swab and/or FCU	TMA SDA	16.4	48	5	3	416	94.1	98.9	90.6*	99.3*	79.3*	0.06*
TMA[39]	≥1 positive result from each reference NAAT; for assay comparison, positive result required from each of other 2 assays	TMA SDA	21.4	30	2	3	166	90.9	98.8	93.8*	98.2*	76.4*	0.09*
SDA[32]	Positive result from ≥2 NAATs with different target regions in urethral swab and/or FCU	TMA SDA	16.4	45	1	7	419	86.5	99.8	97.8*	98.4*	363.5*	0.13*
SDA[39]	≥1 positive result from each reference NAAT; for assay comparison, positive result required from each of other 2 assays	TMA SDA	21.4	31	2	4	178	88.6	98.9	93.9*	97.8*	79.7*	0.12*
SDA[39]	≥1 positive result from each reference NAAT; for assay comparison, positive result required from each of other 2 assays	TMA SDA	21.4	31	2	5	173	86.1	98.9	93.9*	97.2*	75.4*	0.14*
First-catch urine													
TMA[31]	Positive result from ≥1 NAAT in both urethral swab and FCU; or 1 specimen positive on both NAATs	TMA SDA	17.9	94	19	1	638	98.9	98.0†	83.2*	99.8*	34.2*	0.01*
TMA[32]	Positive result from ≥2 NAATs with different target regions in urethral swab and/or FCU	TMA SDA	16.4	50	4	1	417	98.0	99.0	92.6*	99.8*	103.2*	0.02*
TMA[39]	≥1 positive result from each reference NAAT; for assay comparison, positive result required from each of other 2 assays	TMA SDA	21.4	35	0	1	179	97.2	100.0	100.0*	99.4*	Unable to calculate	0.03*
PCR[32]	Positive result from ≥2 NAATs with different target regions in urethral swab and/or FCU	TMA SDA	16.4	51	2	1	418	98.1	99.5	96.2*	99.8*	206.0*	0.02*
SDA[32]	Positive result from ≥2 NAATs with different target regions in urethral swab and/or FCU	TMA SDA	16.4	50	2	2	418	96.2	99.5	96.2*	99.5*	201.9*	0.04*
SDA[39]	≥1 positive result from each reference NAAT; for assay comparison, positive result required from each of other 2 assays	TMA SDA	21.4	35	2	0	178	100.0	98.9	94.6*	100.0*	90.0*	0.00*

Table 8. Diagnostic Accuracy of Nucleic Acid Amplification Tests for Screening for Chlamydia in Men

Test	Definition of a positive screening test	Reference standard	Prevalence (%)	TP (n)	FP (n)	FN (n)	TN (n)	Sens (%)	Spec (%)	PPV (%)	NPV (%)	PLR	NLR
SDA[39]	≥1 positive result from each reference NAAT; for assay comparison, positive result required from each of other 2 assays	TMA SDA	21.4	35	1	1	173	97.2	99.4	97.2*	99.4*	169.2*	0.03*
PCR[36]	≥1 positive result from each reference NAAT	TMA SDA	2.6	29	1	0	1102	100	99.9	96.7	100	1103.0*	0.00*

*Calculated.
†Study reported sensitivity noted above; calculated as 97.1%.

Abbreviations: FCU = first-catch urine; FN = false negative; FP = false positive; n = number; NAAT = nucleic acid amplification test; NLR = negative likelihood ratio; NPV = negative predictive value; PCR = polymerase chain reaction; PLR = positive likelihood ratio; PPV = positive predictive value; SDA = strand displacement assay; Sens = sensitivity; Spec = specificity; TMA = transcription-mediated amplification; TN = true negative; TP = true positive.

Table 9. Summary of Evidence

Main findings from prior USPSTF reviews	Number/type of studies in update	Overall quality*	Limitations	Consistency	Applicability	Summary of findings
Key Question 1. How effective is screening for gonorrhea and chlamydia in reducing complications of infection and transmission or acquisition of disease in asymptomatic, sexually active men and nonpregnant women, including adolescents?						
Chlamydia screening reduced PID in a good-quality RCT (RR, 0.44 [95% CI, 0.20 to 0.90]), but not in a poor-quality RCT (RR, 0.50 [95% CI, 0.23 to 1.08]).	1 good-quality RCT of chlamydia screening in women	Fair	Trial was potentially underpowered; 20% of women were tested outside of the trial. No studies of gonorrhea screening; no studies of chlamydia screening in other populations.	Point estimates consistent with prior trials, although statistical significance varies.	Study conducted in the United Kingdom using self-collected samples.	Screening a subset of asymptomatic young women for chlamydia did not statistically significantly reduce PID over the following year (RR, 0.39 [95% CI, 0.14 to 1.08]); one previous trial reported a reduction.
Key Question 2. How effective are different screening strategies in identifying persons with gonorrhea and chlamydia?						
Nine sets of selective screening criteria for chlamydial infection indicated that age alone had similar or better sensitivity and specificity than more extensive criteria.	1 observational study of chlamydia screening in women	Poor; studies are lacking	No studies of effectiveness, comparing cotesting for concurrent STIs, or evaluating different screening intervals.	NA	Study conducted in the Netherlands with limited applicability to the United States.	A risk prediction tool to identify persons with chlamydia in high-risk populations was not an accurate predictor and may not be relevant to U.S. practice. A previous study indicated that an age cut-off of ≤22 years would identify 80% of cases while testing 50% of women.
Key Question 3. How accurate are screening tests for detecting gonorrhea and chlamydia?						
25 studies of tests for gonorrhea and 33 for chlamydia indicated high accuracy, although studies included symptomatic persons and tests that are no longer used.	10 diagnostic accuracy studies of NAATs	Good	Unclear sampling methods, interpretation of tests, and inclusion of patients with uninterpretable results; some studies had technical shortcomings.	Consistent	Studies included high-prevalence populations (>5%).	Gonorrhea: sensitivity of 91% to 100% and specificity of ≥97% in studies without major limitations. Chlamydia: sensitivity of 86% to 100% and specificity of ≥97% in studies without major limitations. Previous findings are similar, but may not be clinically applicable.
Key Question 4. What are the harms of screening for gonorrhea and chlamydia?						
25 studies of tests for gonorrhea and 33 for chlamydia reported diagnostic accuracy. One qualitative interview study indicated anxiety with a positive test.	10 diagnostic accuracy studies of NAATs	Good for false-positive and false-negative rates; lack of other outcomes	No studies on other harms of screening, such as labeling or anxiety.	Consistent	Studies included high-prevalence populations (>5%).	Gonorrhea: false positive rate of ≤3%; false-negative rate of 0% to 9% in studies without major limitations. Chlamydia: false-positive rate of ≤3%; false-negative rate of 0% to 14% in studies without major limitations. Previous findings are similar, but may not be clinically applicable.
Key Question 1. How effective is screening for gonorrhea and chlamydia in reducing maternal complications, adverse pregnancy and infant outcomes, and transmission or acquisition of disease in asymptomatic pregnant women?						
No studies; prior reviews cited descriptive studies predating the searches.	No studies	NA	NA	NA	NA	NA

Table 9. Summary of Evidence

Main findings from prior USPSTF reviews	Number/type of studies in update	Overall quality*	Limitations	Consistency	Applicability	Summary of findings
Key Question 2. What are the harms of screening for gonorrhea and chlamydia in asymptomatic pregnant women?						
No studies met inclusion criteria.	No studies met inclusion criteria.	NA	NA	NA	NA	

*Overall quality is based on new evidence identified for the update plus previously reviewed evidence.

Abbreviations: CI = confidence interval; NA = not applicable; NAAT = nucleic acid amplification test; PID = pelvic inflammatory disease; RCT = randomized, control trial; RR = relative risk; STI = sexually transmitted infection.

Appendix A. Terminology

Area under receiver operating curve (AUC): Measure of how well a parameter can distinguish between two diagnostic groups.

Enzyme immunoassay (EIA): Assay designed to detect antigens of antibodies by producing an enzyme-triggered color change.

First-catch urine (FCU): Urine sample collected from individuals. Individuals should not have passed urine for at least 3 hours before sample collection. Individual collects first 10 mL of urine.

Indeterminate test result: Test result was not clear.

Negative likelihood ratio (NLR): Ratio between the probability of a negative test result given the presence of the disease and the probability of a negative test result given the absence of the disease.

Negative predictive value (NPV): Proportion of people with a negative test who are free of disease.

Nucleic acid amplification test (NAAT): Nucleic acid amplification tests detect small amounts of DNA or RNA in a test sample by using a series of repeated reactions to make multiple copies of the DNA or RNA that is being detected, thereby amplifying the signal from that piece of DNA or RNA. Several different categories exist, including:

- Transcription-mediated amplification (TMA)
- Strand displacement amplification (SDA)
- Polymerase chain reaction (PCR)
- Ligase chain reaction (LCR)

Number needed to invite (NNI): Average number of people who need to be invited to screen to find one positive case of disease/infection.

Number needed to screen (NNS): Average number of people who need to be screened to find one positive case of disease/infection.

Positive likelihood ratio (PLR): Ratio between the probability of a positive test result given the presence of the disease and the probability of a positive test result given the absence of the disease.

Positive predictive value (PPV): Proportion of people with a positive test who have the disease.

Relative risk (RR): Ratio of the risk of an event among an exposed population to the risk among the unexposed.

Sensitivity: Proportion of truly diseased/infected persons in the screened population who are identified as diseased by the screening test—that is, the true-positive rate.

Appendix A. Terminology

<u>Specificity:</u> Proportion of truly nondiseased/noninfected persons who are identified as such by the screening test—that is, the true-negative rate.

Screening in Pregnant Women: Maternal and Neonatal Outcomes
Database: Ovid MEDLINE(R) without Revisions
Search Strategy:
----
1   exp GONORRHEA/
2   exp NEISSERIA GONORRHOEAE/
3   gonorrh$.mp. [mp=title, abstract, original title, name of substance word, subject heading word, protocol supplementary concept, rare disease supplementary concept, unique identifier]
4   1 or 2 or 3
5   exp mass screening/ or screen$.mp.
6   4 and 5
7   exp GONORRHEA/di
8   6 or 7
9   neonat$.mp. or exp Infant, Newborn/
10 8 and 9
11 maternal fetal transmission.mp. or exp Disease Transmission, Vertical/
12 exp GONORRHEA/tm [Transmission]
13 4 and 11
14 7 and 11
15 9 and 12
16 13 or 15
17 limit 16 to human
18 10 or 17

Risks
Database: Ovid MEDLINE(R) without Revisions
Search Strategy:
----
1   exp gonorrhea/
2   exp Neisseria gonorrhoeae/
3   1 or 2
4   exp Risk/
5   exp Risk Reduction Behavior/
6   exp Risk-Taking/
7   exp Risk Management/
8   4 or 5 or 6 or 7
9   3 or 8

Database: EBM Reviews – Cochrane Central Register of Controlled Trials
Search Strategy:
----
1   gonorrh$.mp. [mp=title, original title, abstract, mesh headings, heading words, keyword]
2   risk$.mp. [mp=title, original title, abstract, mesh headings, heading words, keyword]
3   1 and 2

Appendix B1. Search Strategies

Test Performance
Database: Ovid MEDLINE(R) without Revisions
Search Strategy:

----

1   exp gonorrhea/
2   exp Neisseria gonorrhoeae/
3   1 or 2
4   exp "Sensitivity and Specificity"/
5   exp Diagnostic Errors/
6   4 or 5
7   3 and 6

Database: EBM Reviews – Cochrane Central Register of Controlled Trials
Search Strategy:

----

1   gonorrh$.mp. [mp=title, original title, abstract, mesh headings, heading words, keyword]
2   (sensitiv$ or accurate$ or accuracy or predict$ or misdiagnos$ or misinterpret$ or ((diagnos$ or detect$ or discover$) adj5 (error$ or erroneous$ or fail$ or bias$)) or (false$ adj3 (positiv$ or negativ$))).mp. [mp=title, original title, abstract, mesh headings, heading words, keyword]
3   1 and 2

Searches Conducted for Chlamydia Only

Overall
Database: EBM Reviews – Cochrane Central Register of Controlled Trials
Search Strategy:

----

1   chlamyd$.mp. [mp=title, original title, abstract, mesh headings, heading words, keyword]
2   risk$.mp. [mp=title, original title, abstract, mesh headings, heading words, keyword]
3   1 and 2
4   screen$.mp. [mp=title, original title, abstract, mesh headings, heading words, keyword]
5   1 and 4
6   (sensitiv$ or accurate$ or accuracy or predict$ or misdiagnos$ or misinterpret$ or ((diagnos$ or detect$ or discover$) adj5 (error$ or erroneous$ or fail$ or bias$)) or (false$ adj3 (positiv$ or negativ$))).mp. [mp=title, original title, abstract, mesh headings, heading words, keyword]
7   1 and 6
8   3 or 5 or 7

Database: EBM Reviews – Cochrane Database of Systematic Reviews
Search Strategy:

----

1   chlamyd$.mp. [mp=title, abstract, full text, keywords, caption text]
2   risk$.mp. [mp=title, abstract, full text, keywords, caption text]
3   1 and 2
4   screen$.mp. [mp=title, abstract, full text, keywords, caption text]
5   1 and 4

6   (sensitiv$ or accurate$ or accuracy or predict$ or misdiagnos$ or misinterpret$ or ((diagnos$ or detect$ or discover$) adj5 (error$ or erroneous$ or fail$ or bias$)) or (false$ adj3 (positiv$ or negativ$))).mp. [mp=title, abstract, full text, keywords, caption text]
7   1 and 6
8   3 or 5 or 7

Database: EBM Reviews – Database of Abstracts of Reviews of Effects
Search Strategy:
----
1   chlamyd$.mp. [mp=title, full text, keywords]
2   (cost or costs or costing or fund or funding or funded or economic$ or expenditur$ or insuran$ or dollar$).mp. [mp=title, full text, keywords]
3   1 and 2
4   risk$.mp. [mp=title, full text, keywords]
5   1 and 4
6   screen$.mp. [mp=title, full text, keywords]
7   1 and 6
8   (sensitiv$ or accurate$ or accuracy or predict$ or misdiagnos$ or misinterpret$ or ((diagnos$ or detect$ or discover$) adj5 (error$ or erroneous$ or fail$ or bias$)) or (false$ adj3 (positiv$ or negativ$))).mp. [mp=title, full text, keywords]
9   1 and 8
10   3 or 5 or 7 or 9

Database: EBM Reviews – Health Technology Assessment
Search Strategy:
----
1   chlamyd$.mp. [mp=title, text, subject heading word]
2   risk$.mp. [mp=title, text, subject heading word]
3   1 and 2
4   screen$.mp. [mp=title, text, subject heading word]
5   1 and 4
6   (sensitiv$ or accurate$ or accuracy or predict$ or misdiagnos$ or misinterpret$ or ((diagnos$ or detect$ or discover$) adj5 (error$ or erroneous$ or fail$ or bias$)) or (false$ adj3 (positiv$ or negativ$))).mp. [mp=title, text, subject heading word]
7   1 and 6
8   3 or 5 or 7

Screening
Database: Ovid MEDLINE(R) without Revisions
Search Strategy:
----
1   exp chlamydia infections/
2   exp chlamydia trachomatis/
3   1 or 2
4   exp Mass Screening/
5   3 and 4

Appendix B1. Search Strategies

Database: EBM Reviews – Cochrane Central Register of Controlled Trials
Search Strategy:
----
1   chlamyd$.mp. [mp=title, original title, abstract, mesh headings, heading words, keyword]
2   screen$.mp. [mp=title, original title, abstract, mesh headings, heading words, keyword]
3   1 and 2

Screening in Pregnant Women – Maternal Outcomes

Database: Ovid MEDLINE(R) without Revisions
Search Strategy:
----
1   exp chlamydia infections/
2   exp chlamydia trachomatis/
3   1 or 2
4   exp mass screening/ or screen$.mp.
5   3 and 4
6   exp chlamydia infections/di
7   5 or 6
8   exp PREGNANCY/ or exp PREGNANCY COMPLICATIONS/
9   (septic$ adj3 abort$).mp. [mp=title, abstract, original title, name of substance word, subject heading word, protocol supplementary concept, rare disease supplementary concept, unique identifier]
10   exp Fetal Death/
11   (stillborn or stillbirth$).mp. [mp=title, abstract, original title, name of substance word, subject heading word, protocol supplementary concept, rare disease supplementary concept, unique identifier]
12   (preterm$ or prematur$).mp. [mp=title, abstract, original title, name of substance word, subject heading word, protocol supplementary concept, rare disease supplementary concept, unique identifier]
13   exp Infant, Low Birth Weight/
14   (low adj3 birth weight$).mp. [mp=title, abstract, original title, name of substance word, subject heading word, protocol supplementary concept, rare disease supplementary concept, unique identifier]
15   ((low or lower$ or reduc$) adj3 (weight$ or birthweight$)).mp. [mp=title, abstract, original title, name of substance word, subject heading word, protocol supplementary concept, rare disease supplementary concept, unique identifier]
16   chorioamnionit$.mp. [mp=title, abstract, original title, name of substance word, subject heading word, protocol supplementary concept, rare disease supplementary concept, unique identifier]
17   9 or 10 or 11 or 12 or 13 or 14 or 15 or 16
18   7 and 17

Screening in Pregnant Women – Neonatal Outcomes

Database: Ovid MEDLINE(R) without Revisions
Search Strategy:

Appendix B1. Search Strategies

1   exp chlamydia infections/
2   exp chlamydia trachomatis/
3   1 or 2
4   exp mass screening/ or screen$.mp.
5   3 and 4
6   exp chlamydia infections/di
7   5 or 6
8   neonat$.mp. or exp Infant, Newborn/
9   7 and 8
10   maternal fetal transmission.mp. or exp Disease Transmission, Vertical/
11   exp chlamydia infection/tm
12   7 and 10
13   8 and 11
14   12 or 13
15   limit 14 to human

Risks
Database: Ovid MEDLINE(R) without Revisions
Search Strategy:
----
1   exp chlamydia infections/
2   exp chlamydia trachomatis/
3   1 or 2
4   exp Risk/
5   exp Risk Reduction Behavior/
6   exp Risk-Taking/
7   exp Risk Management/
8   8 or 9 or 10 or 11
9   3 and 12

Database: EBM Reviews – Cochrane Central Register of Controlled Trials
Search Strategy:
----
1   chlamyd$.mp. [mp=title, original title, abstract, mesh headings, heading words, keyword]
2   risk$.mp. [mp=title, original title, abstract, mesh headings, heading words, keyword]
3   1 and 2

Test Performance
Database: Ovid MEDLINE(R) without Revisions
Search Strategy:
----
1   exp chlamydia infections/
2   exp chlamydia trachomatis/
3   1 or 2
4   exp "Sensitivity and Specificity"/
5   exp Diagnostic Errors/

6   4 or 5
7   3 and 6

Database: EBM Reviews – Cochrane Central Register of Controlled Trials
Search Strategy:
----
1   chlamyd$.mp. [mp=title, original title, abstract, mesh headings, heading words, keyword]
2   (sensitiv$ or accurate$ or accuracy or predict$ or misdiagnos$ or misinterpret$ or ((diagnos$ or detect$ or discover$) adj5 (error$ or erroneous$ or fail$ or bias$)) or (false$ adj3 (positiv$ or negativ$))).mp. [mp=title, original title, abstract, mesh headings, heading words, keyword]
3   1 and 2

Appendix B2. Inclusion and Exclusion Criteria

	Include	Exclude
Population	Asymptomatic, sexually active men and women (pregnant and nonpregnant), including adolescents	Symptomatic patients, children age <13 years, persons with other STIs
Interventions	Nonpregnant population: Screening effectiveness; screening strategies to detect infection, including selective screening of high-risk groups, sampling from various anatomical sites, cotesting for concurrent STIs, and use of different screening intervals; tests that detect chlamydia or gonorrhea in biological specimens from various anatomical sites (urine, endocervix, urethra, vagina, anus, pharynx) Pregnant population: Screening effectiveness	Tests that are not approved by the FDA
Outcomes	Nonpregnant population: Reduction in pelvic inflammatory disease, ectopic pregnancy, infertility, chronic pelvic pain, disease transmission, epididymitis, and other clinical outcomes; detection of infection and diagnostic accuracy; and harms from screening, such as labeling and false-negative or false-positive results Pregnant population: Reduction in disease transmission, preterm birth, neonatal clinical outcomes, and other pregnancy clinical outcomes	Intermediate outcomes
Study types and designs	All key questions: Good quality systematic reviews Benefits: Randomized, control trials; controlled observational trials Harms: Randomized, control trials; controlled observational trials; and uncontrolled observational trials	Benefits: Uncontrolled observational trials, case studies Harms: Small uncontrolled observational trials, case studies

Abbreviations: FDA = U.S. Food and Drug Administration; STI = sexually transmitted infection.

Appendix B3. Literature Flow Diagram

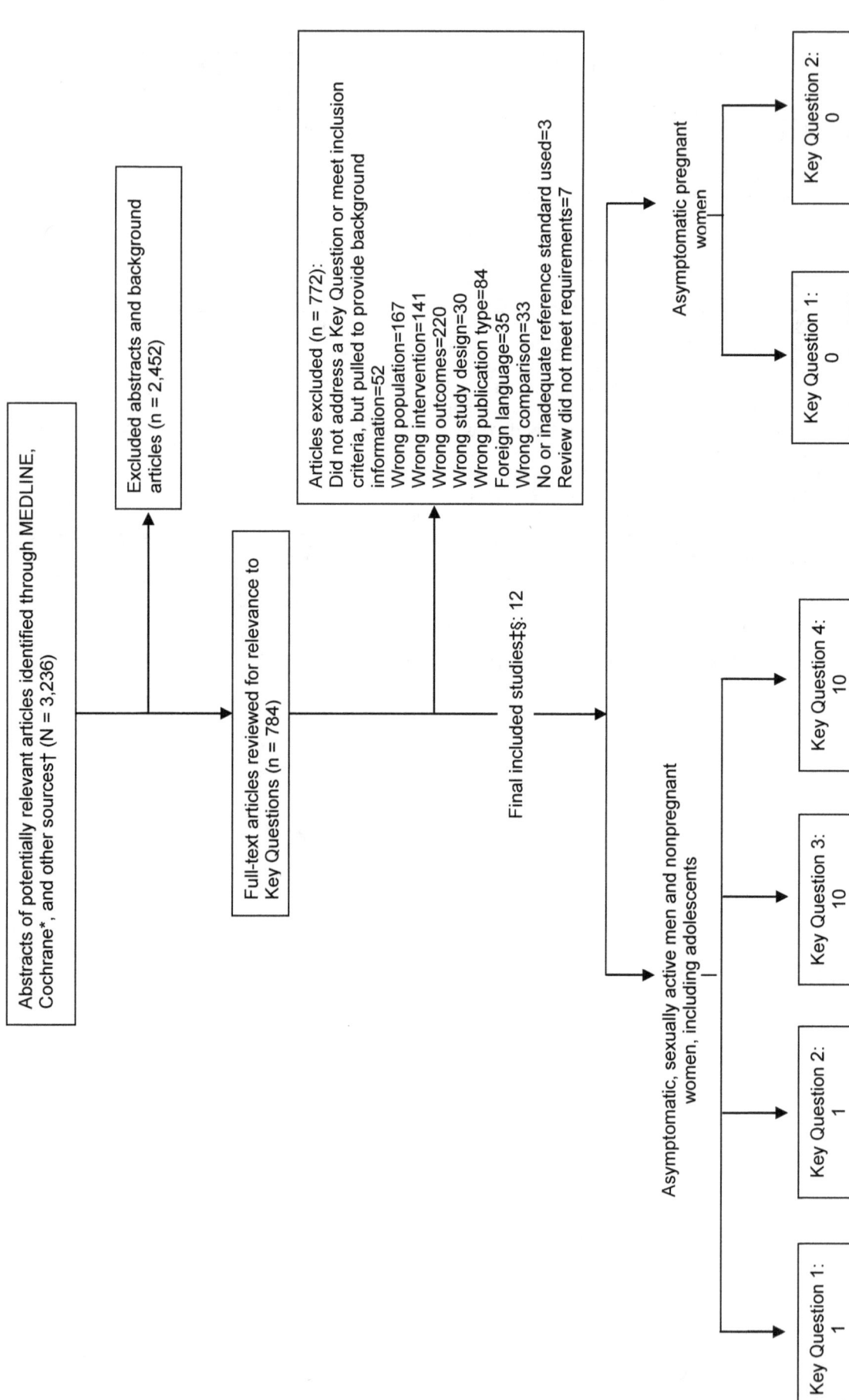

Abstracts of potentially relevant articles identified through MEDLINE, Cochrane*, and other sources† (N = 3,236)

Excluded abstracts and background articles (n = 2,452)

Full-text articles reviewed for relevance to Key Questions (n = 784)

Articles excluded (n = 772):
Did not address a Key Question or meet inclusion criteria, but pulled to provide background information=52
Wrong population=167
Wrong intervention=141
Wrong outcomes=220
Wrong study design=30
Wrong publication type=84
Foreign language=35
Wrong comparison=33
No or inadequate reference standard used=3
Review did not meet requirements=7

Final included studies‡§: 12

Asymptomatic, sexually active men and nonpregnant women, including adolescents

Key Question 1: 1

Key Question 2: 1

Key Question 3: 10

Key Question 4: 10

Asymptomatic pregnant women

Key Question 1: 0

Key Question 2: 0

*Cochrane databases include the Cochrane Central Register of Controlled Trials and the Cochrane Database of Systematic Reviews.
†Identified from reference lists, hand searching, and suggestions from experts.
‡Studies that provided data and contributed to the body of evidence were considered "included."
§Studies may have provided data for more than one Key Question.

Appendix B4. Excluded Studies

Key to exclusion codes

2	Excluded because it does not address a Key Question or meet inclusion criteria, but pulled to provide background information
3	Wrong population
4	Wrong intervention
5	Wrong outcomes
6	Wrong study design for Key Question
7	Wrong publication type
8	Foreign language
9	Appears in an included systematic review, no original data
10	Wrong comparison
11	No or inadequate reference standard used
12	Review did not meet our requirements

Molecular Diagnostics: LCR, the ligase chain reaction. 2003; http://chlamydiae.com/twiki/bin/view/Diagnostics/LcrTest. Accessed 22 May, 2013Exclusion code: 2.

Adderley-Kelly B, Stephens EM. Chlamydia: A major health threat to adolescents and young adults. *Abnf J.* 2005;16(3):52-55
Exclusion code: 6

Aghaizu A, Adams EJ, Turner K, et al. What is the cost of pelvic inflammatory disease and how much could be prevented by screening for chlamydia trachomatis? Cost analysis of the Prevention of Pelvic Infection (POPI) trial. *Sex Transm Infect.* 2011;87(4):312-317
Exclusion code: 5

Agrawal T, Vats V, Salhan S, Mittal A. Local markers for prediction of women at higher risk of developing sequelae to Chlamydia trachomatis infection. *Am J Reprod Immunol.* 2007;57(2):153-159
Exclusion code: 5

Akande V, Turner C, Horner P, Horne A, Pacey A, British Fertility S. Impact of Chlamydia trachomatis in the reproductive setting: British Fertility Society Guidelines for practice. *Hum Fertil (Camb).* 2010;13(3):115-125
Exclusion code: 6

Alary M, Poulin C, Bouchard C, et al. Evaluation of a modified sanitary napkin as a sample self-collection device for the detection of genital chlamydial infection in women. *J Clin Microbiol.* 2001;39(7):2508-2512
Exclusion code: 4

Aldeen T, Jacobs J, Powell R. Screening university students for genital chlamydial infection: another lesson to learn. *Sex Health.* 2010;7(4):491-494
Exclusion code: 5

Alexander S, Ison C. Evaluation of commercial kits for the identification of Neisseria gonorrhoeae. *J Med Microbiol.* 2005;54(Pt 9):827-831
Exclusion code: 10

Alexander S, Ison C, Parry J, et al. Self-taken pharyngeal and rectal swabs are appropriate for the detection of Chlamydia trachomatis and Neisseria gonorrhoeae in asymptomatic men who have sex with men. *Sex Transm Infect.* 2008;84(6):488-492
Exclusion code: 4

Alexander S, Martin I, Ison C. Confirming the Chlamydia trachomatis status of referred rectal specimens. *Sex Transm Infect.* 2007;83(4):327-329
Exclusion code: 5

Al-Tayyib AA, Miller WC, Rogers SM, et al. Evaluation of risk score algorithms for detection of chlamydial and gonococcal infections in an emergency department setting. *Acad Emerg Med.* 2008;15(2):126-135
Exclusion code: 10

Althaus CL, Heijne JCM, Roellin A, Low N. Transmission dynamics of Chlamydia trachomatis affect the impact of screening programmes. *Epidemics.* 2010;2(3):123-131
Exclusion code: 6

American Academy of Family Physicians. USPSTF Screening for Chlamydial Infection: Recommendation Statement. 2007; http://www.aafp.org/afp/2007/1201/p1695.html. Accessed 5 Dec, 2012
Exclusion code: 2.

Appendix B4. Excluded Studies

American Academy of Pediatrics. What's new with 2010 STD treatment guidelines from the CDC? 2011; http://aapnews.aappublications.org/content/32/2/7.full. Accessed 5 Dec, 2012
Exclusion code: 2.

American College of Obstetricians and Gynecologists. Committee opinion no. 506: expedited partner therapy in the management of gonorrhea and chlamydia by obstetrician-gynecologists. *Obstet Gynecol.* 2011;118(3):761-766
Exclusion code: 7

American College of Physicians. ACP Pocket Guide to Selected Preventive Services for Adults: Gonorrhea. 2012; http://www.acponline.org/mobile/cyppocketguide/gonorrhea_screening.html. Accessed 5 Dec, 2012
Exclusion code: 2.

American College of Physicians. ACP Pocket Guide to Selected Preventive Services for Adults: Chlamydia. 2012; http://www.acponline.org/mobile/cyppocketguide/chlamydia_screening.html. Accessed 5 Dec 2012
Exclusion code: 2.

American Medical Association, Moyer CS. STDs increasing among young women; more prevention urged. 2009; http://www.ama-assn.org/amednews/2009/12/07/prsb1207.htm. Accessed 5 Dec, 2012
Exclusion code: 2.

Amortegui AJ, Meyer MP. Enzyme immunoassay for detection of Chlamydia trachomatis from the cervix. *Obstet Gynecol.* 1985;65(4):523-526
Exclusion code: 4

Anagrius C, Mjornberg P-A. [Gathering round the Chlamydia infection problems: tests and contact tracing necessary--changed sexual behavior is also needed!]. *Lakartidningen.* 2006;103(28-29):2158; discussion 2160-2151
Exclusion code: 8

Andersen B, Gundgaard J, Kretzschmar M, Olsen J, Welte R, Oster-Gaard L. Prediction of costs, effectiveness, and disease control of a population-based program using home sampling for diagnosis of urogenital Chlamydia trachomatis Infections. *Sex Transm Dis.* 2006;33(7):407-415
Exclusion code: 3

Andersen B, Olesen F. Screening for Chlamydia trachomatis. *BMJ.* 2012;345:e4231

Exclusion code: 7

Andersen B, Olesen F, Moller JK, Ostergaard L. Population-based strategies for outreach screening of urogenital Chlamydia trachomatis infections: a randomized, controlled trial. *J Infect Dis.* 2002;185(2):252-258
Exclusion code: 3

Andersen B, Ostergaard L, Olesen F. [Lack of evidence to support chlamydia infection screening]. *Ugeskr Laeger.* 2010;172(28):2059-2061
Exclusion code: 7

Andersen B, Ostergaard L, Puho E, Skriver MV, Schonheyder HC. Ectopic pregnancies and reproductive capacity after Chlamydia trachomatis positive and negative test results: a historical follow-up study. *Sex Transm Dis.* 2005;32(6):377-381
Exclusion code: 4

Andersen B, Ostergaard L, Thomsen RW, Schonheyder H. Chlamydia trachomatis infection and risk of ectopic pregnancy. *Sex Transm Dis.* 2007;34(1):59; author reply 60
Exclusion code: 7

Andersen B, van Valkengoed I, Sokolowski I, Moller JK, Ostergaard L, Olesen F. Impact of intensified testing for urogenital Chlamydia trachomatis infections: a randomised study with 9-year follow-up. *Sex Transm Infect.* 2011;87(2):156-161
Exclusion code: 3

Anderson C, Thornley T. A pharmacy-based private chlamydia screening programme: results from the first 2 years of screening and treatment. *Int J Clin Pharm.* 2011;33(1):88-91
Exclusion code: 4

Andrews WW, Klebanoff MA, Thom EA, et al. Midpregnancy genitourinary tract infection with Chlamydia trachomatis: association with subsequent preterm delivery in women with bacterial vaginosis and Trichomonas vaginalis. *Am J Obstet Gynecol.* 2006;194(2):493-500
Exclusion code: 5

Angles d'Auriac M, Refseth UH, Espelund M, Moi H, Storvold G, Jeansson S. A new automated method for isolation of Chlamydia trachomatis from urine eliminates inhibition and increases robustness for NAAT systems. *J Microbiol Methods.* 2007;70(3):416-423
Exclusion code: 4

Appendix B4. Excluded Studies

Annan NT, Sullivan AK, Nori A, et al. Rectal chlamydia--a reservoir of undiagnosed infection in men who have sex with men. *Sex Transm Infect.* 2009;85(3):176-179
Exclusion code: 10

Anschuetz GL, Asbel L, Spain CV, et al. Association between enhanced screening for Chlamydia trachomatis and Neisseria gonorrhoeae and reductions in sequelae among women. *J Adolesc Health.* 2012;51(1):80-85
Exclusion code: 10

Anttila T, Tenkanen L, Lumme S, et al. Chlamydial antibodies and risk of prostate cancer. *Cancer Epidemiol Biomarkers Prev.* 2005;14(2):385-389
Exclusion code: 6

Arcari CM, Gaydos JC, Howell MR, McKee KT, Gaydos CA. Feasibility and short-term impact of linked education and urine screening interventions for Chlamydia and gonorrhea in male army recruits. *Sex Transm Dis.* 2004;31(7):443-447
Exclusion code: 4

Arustamian KK. [Risk factors of urogenital chlamydiosis in women of reproductive age]. *Georgian Med.* 2006(139):76-78
Exclusion code: 8

Arustamian KK. [Comparative analysis of methods for diagnostics of chlamydial infection in women of reproductive age]. *Georgian Med.* 2006(139):73-75
Exclusion code: 8

Arya R, Mannion PT, Woodcock K, Haddad NG. Incidence of genital Chlamydia trachomatis infection in the male partners attending an infertility clinic. *J Obstet Gynaecol.* 2005;25(4):364-366
Exclusion code: 2

Asbel LE, Newbern EC, Salmon M, Spain CV, Goldberg M. School-based screening for Chlamydia trachomatis and Neisseria gonorrhoeae among Philadelphia public high school students. *Sex Transm Dis.* 2006;33(10):614-620
Exclusion code: 10

Atherton H, Oakeshott P, Aghaizu A, Hay P, Kerry S. Use of an online questionnaire for follow-up of young female students recruited to a randomised controlled trial of chlamydia screening. *J Epidemiol Community Health.* 2010;64(7):580-584
Exclusion code: 4

Auerswald CL, Sugano E, Ellen JM, Klausner JD. Street-based STD testing and treatment of homeless youth are feasible, acceptable and effective. *J Adolesc Health.* 2006;38(3):208-212
Exclusion code: 10

Azariah S, McKernon S, Werder S. Large increase in opportunistic testing for chlamydia during a pilot project in a primary health organisation. *J Prim Health Care.* 2013;5(2):141-145
Exclusion code: 6

Bachmann LH, Johnson RE, Cheng H, et al. Nucleic acid amplification tests for diagnosis of Neisseria gonorrhoeae and Chlamydia trachomatis rectal infections. *J Clin Microbiol.* 2010;48(5):1827-1832
Exclusion code: 3

Bachmann LH, Johnson RE, Cheng H, Markowitz LE, Papp JR, Hook EW, 3rd. Nucleic acid amplification tests for diagnosis of Neisseria gonorrhoeae oropharyngeal infections. *J Clin Microbiol.* 2009;47(4):902-907
Exclusion code: 3

Bacon L. Chlamydia testing in contraceptive clinics: who, where, how and why? *J Fam Plann Reprod Health Care.* 2004;30(2):82-83
Exclusion code: 7

Baeten JM, Overbaugh J. Measuring the infectiousness of persons with HIV-1: opportunities for preventing sexual HIV-1 transmission. *Curr HIV Res.* 2003;1(1):69-86
Exclusion code: 2

Bakken IJ. Chlamydia trachomatis and ectopic pregnancy: recent epidemiological findings. *Curr Opin Infect Dis.* 2008;21(1):77-82
Exclusion code: 6

Bakken IJ, Bratt H, Skjeldestad FE, Nordbo SA. [Detection of chlamydia trachomatis in urine, vulval and cervical swabs]. *Tidsskr Nor Laegeforen.* 2005;125(12):1629-1630
Exclusion code: 8

Bakken IJ, Ghaderi S. Incidence of pelvic inflammatory disease in a large cohort of women tested for Chlamydia trachomatis: a historical follow-up study. *BMC Infect Dis.* 2009;9:130
Exclusion code: 6

Bakken IJ, Skjeldestad FE, Halvorsen TF, Thomassen T, Storvold G, Nordbo SA. Chlamydia trachomatis among young Norwegian men: sexual

Appendix B4. Excluded Studies

behavior and genitourinary symptoms. *Sex Transm Dis.* 2007;34(4):245-249
Exclusion code: 6

Bakken IJ, Skjeldestad FE, Lydersen S, Nordbo SA. Births and ectopic pregnancies in a large cohort of women tested for Chlamydia trachomatis. *Sex Transm Dis.* 2007;34(10):739-743
Exclusion code: 3

Bakken IJ, Skjeldestad FE, Nordbo SA. Chlamydia trachomatis infections increase the risk for ectopic pregnancy: a population-based, nested case-control study. *Sex Transm Dis.* 2007;34(3):166-169
Exclusion code: 3

Bakken IJ, Skjeldestad FE, Overness T, Nordbo SA, Storvold G. [Chlamydia infections and sexual behavior among young women]. *Tidsskr Nor Laegeforen.* 2004;124(12):1633-1635
Exclusion code: 8

Baldwin SB, Djambazov B, Papenfuss M, et al. Chlamydial infection in women along the US-Mexico border. *Int J STD AIDS.* 2004;15(12):815-821
Exclusion code: 5

Balfe M, Brugha R, O'Connell E, Vaughan D, O'Donovan D. Men's attitudes towards chlamydia screening: a narrative review. *Sex Health.* 2012;9(2):120-130
Exclusion code: 5

Balla E. [Chlamydia trachomatis infections in neonates--overview of current laboratory diagnostics]. *Orv Hetil.* 2009;150(17):805-809
Exclusion code: 8

Bandea CI, Koumans EH, Sawyer MK, et al. Evaluation of the rapid BioStar optical immunoassay for detection of Chlamydia trachomatis in adolescent women. *J Clin Microbiol.* 2009;47(1):215-216
Exclusion code: 4

Bangor-Jones RD. Sexual health in general practice: do practitioners comply with the sexually transmitted infections guidelines for management of suspected chlamydial infections? *Int J STD AIDS.* 2011;22(9):523-524
Exclusion code: 3

Barabasi Z. [Treatment of conjunctivitis]. *Orv Hetil.* 2004;145(41):2107-2110
Exclusion code: 8

Baraitser P, Alexander S, Sheringham J. Chlamydia trachomatis screening in young women. *Curr Opin Obstet Gynecol.* 2011;23(5):315-320
Exclusion code: 7

Barbee L, Dombrowski JC, Kerani R, Golden MR. Effect of nucleic acid amplification testing on detection of extragenital gonorrhea and chlamydial infections in men who have sex with men sexually transmitted disease clinic patients. *Sex Transm Dis.* 2014;41(3):168-172
Exclusion code: 4

Barry PM, Kent CK, Klausner JD. Risk factors for gonorrhea among heterosexuals--San Francisco, 2006. *Sex Transm Dis.* 2009;36(2 Suppl):S62-66
Exclusion code: 5

Barry PM, Kent CK, Philip SS, Klausner JD. Results of a program to test women for rectal chlamydia and gonorrhea. *Obstet Gynecol.* 2010;115(4):753-759
Exclusion code: 3

Barry PM, Kent CK, Scott KC, Goldenson J, Klausner JD. Is jail screening associated with a decrease in Chlamydia positivity among females seeking health services at community clinics?-San Francisco, 1997-2004. *Sex Transm Dis.* 2009;36(2 Suppl):S22-28
Exclusion code: 10

Barry PM, Kent CK, Scott KC, Snell A, Goldenson J, Klausner JD. Optimising sexually transmitted infection screening in correctional facilities: San Francisco, 2003-2005. *Sex Transm Infect.* 2007;83(5):416-418
Exclusion code: 10

Barry PM, Scott KC, McCright J, et al. Stay in school? Results of a sexually transmitted diseases screening program in San Francisco high schools-2007. *Sex Transm Dis.* 2008;35(6):550-552
Exclusion code: 10

Baseviciene I, Sumskas L. [Use of contraceptives among adolescent girls and its relation with the Chlamydia trachomatis infection]. *Medicina (Kaunas).* 2004;40(10):997-1003
Exclusion code: 5

Baud D, Regan L, Greub G. Comparison of five commercial serological tests for the detection of anti-Chlamydia trachomatis antibodies. *Eur J Clin Microbiol Infect Dis.* 2010;29(6):669-675
Exclusion code: 4

Appendix B4. Excluded Studies

Beebe JL, Masters H, Jungkind D, Heltzel DM, Weinberg A. Confirmation of the Syva MicroTrak enzyme immunoassay for chlamydia trachomatis by Syva Direct Fluorescent Antibody Test. *Sex Transm Dis.* 1996;23(6):465-470
Exclusion code: 3

Bekler C, Kultursay N, Ozacar T, Sayiner A, Yalaz M, Akisu M. Chlamydial infections in term and preterm neonates. *Jpn J Infect Dis.* 2012;65(1):1-6
Exclusion code: 3

Benn PD, Rooney G, Carder C, et al. Chlamydia trachomatis and Neisseria gonorrhoeae infection and the sexual behaviour of men who have sex with men. *Sex Transm Infect.* 2007;83(2):106-112
Exclusion code: 3

Benzaken AS, Galban EG, Antunes W, et al. Diagnosis of gonococcal infection in high risk women using a rapid test. *Sex Transm Infect.* 2006;82 Suppl 5:v26-28
Exclusion code: 4

Berger RE. Comparison of three nucleic acid amplification tests for detection of Chlamydia trachomatis in urine specimens. *J Urol.* 2005;173(6):1989-1990
Exclusion code: 7

Berger RE. Comparison of first void urine and urogenital swab specimens for detection of Mycoplasma genitalium and Chlamydia trachomatis by polymerase chain reaction in patients attending a sexually transmitted disease clinic. *J Urol.* 2005;173(6):1989-1990
Exclusion code: 7

Berman SM, Satterwhite CL. A paradox: overscreening of older women for Chlamydia while too few younger women are being tested. *Sex Transm Dis.* 2011;38(2):130-132
Exclusion code: 7

Bernstein KT, Marcus JL, Nieri G, Philip SS, Klausner JD. Rectal gonorrhea and chlamydia reinfection is associated with increased risk of HIV seroconversion. *J Acquir Immune Defic Syndr.* 2010;53(4):537-543
Exclusion code: 5

Bernstein KT, Marcus JL, Snell A, Liska S, Rauch L, Philip SS. Reduction in unnecessary Chlamydia screening among older women at title X-funded family planning sites following a structural intervention--San Francisco, 2009. *Sex Transm Dis.* 2011;38(2):127-129
Exclusion code: 6

Bernstein KT, Mehta SD, Rompalo AM, Erbelding EJ. Cost-effectiveness of screening strategies for Gonorrhea among females in private sector care. *Obstet Gynecol.* 2006;107(4):813-821
Exclusion code: 6

Berry SA, Ghanem KG, Page KR, et al. Increased gonorrhoea and chlamydia testing did not increase case detection in an HIV clinical cohort 1999-2007. *Sex Transm Infect.* 2011;87(6):469-475
Exclusion code: 3

Berwald N, Cheng S, Augenbraun M, Abu-Lawi K, Lucchesi M, Zehtabchi S. Self-administered vaginal swabs are a feasible alternative to physician-assisted cervical swabs for sexually transmitted infection screening in the emergency department. *Acad Emerg Med.* 2009;16(4):360-363
Exclusion code: 3

Bhalla P, Baveja UK, Chawla R, et al. Simultaneous detection of Neisseria gonorrhoeae and Chlamydia trachomatis by PCR in genitourinary specimens from men and women attending an STD clinic. *J Commun Dis.* 2007;39(1):1-6
Exclusion code: 3

Bialasiewicz S, Whiley DM, Buhrer-Skinner M, et al. A novel gel-based method for self-collection and ambient temperature postal transport of urine for PCR detection of Chlamydia trachomatis. *Sex Transm Infect.* 2009;85(2):102-105
Exclusion code: 4

Bielecki R, Zdrodowska-Stefanow B, Ostaszewska-Puchalska I, Kozlowski R, Pucilo K. [Role of Chlamydia trachomatis infection in the pathology of male urogenital tract]. *Przegl Lek.* 2004;61(3):170-176
Exclusion code: 8

Bignell C, Ison CA, Jungmann E. Gonorrhoea. *Sex Transm Infect.* 2006;82 Suppl 4:iv6-9
Exclusion code: 7

Bilardi JE, Sanci LA, Fairley CK, et al. The experience of providing young people attending general practice with an online risk assessment tool to assess their own sexual health risk. *BMC Infect Dis.* 2009;9:29
Exclusion code: 5

Appendix B4. Excluded Studies

Biro FM, Reising SF, Doughman JA, Kollar LM, Rosenthal SL. A comparison of diagnostic methods in adolescent girls with and without symptoms of Chlamydia urogenital infection. *Pediatrics.* 1994;93(3):476-480
Exclusion code: 4

Biros E, Bodnar J, Biros I, et al. Nucleic acid amplification technique for detection of Chlamydia trachomatis infection from clinical urogenital swabs. *Folia Microbiol (Praha).* 2007;52(4):437-442
Exclusion code: 4

Bissessor M, Tabrizi SN, Fairley CK, et al. Differing Neisseria gonorrhoeae bacterial loads in the pharynx and rectum in men who have sex with men: Implications for gonococcal detection, transmission, and control. *J Clin Microbiol.* 2011;49(12):4304-4306
Exclusion code: 2

Bjartling C, Persson K. [Chlamydia and genital mycoplasma: epidemiology and risks]. *Lakartidningen.* 2010;107(6):341-345
Exclusion code: 8

Blake DR. Approaches to Chlamydia screening: one size does not fit all. *Arch Pediatr Adolesc Med.* 2009;163(6):585-586
Exclusion code: 7

Blake DR, Lemay CA, Gaydos CA, Quinn TC. Performance of urine leukocyte esterase in asymptomatic male youth: another look with nucleic acid amplification testing as the gold standard for Chlamydia detection. *J Adolesc Health.* 2005;36(4):337-341
Exclusion code: 4

Blas MM, Canchihuaman FA, Alva IE, Hawes SE. Pregnancy outcomes in women infected with Chlamydia trachomatis: a population-based cohort study in Washington State. *Sex Transm Infect.* 2007;83(4):314-318
Exclusion code: 5

Blatt AJ, Lieberman JM, Hoover DR, Kaufman HW. Chlamydial and gonococcal testing during pregnancy in the United States. *Am J Obstet Gynecol.* 2012;207(1):55.e51-58
Exclusion code: 5

Bloom MS, Hu Z, Gaydos JC, Brundage JF, Tobler SK. Incidence rates of pelvic inflammatory disease diagnoses among Army and Navy recruits potential

impacts of Chlamydia screening policies. *Am J Prev Med.* 2008;34(6):471-477
Exclusion code: 5

Boeke AJP, van Bergen JEAM, Morre SA, van Everdingen JJE. [The risk of pelvic inflammatory disease associated with urogenital infection with Chlamydia trachomatis; literature review]. *Ned Tijdschr Geneeskd.* 2005;149(16):878-884
Exclusion code: 8

Boel CHE, van Herk CMC, Berretty PJM, Onland GHW, van den Brule AJC. Evaluation of conventional and real-time PCR assays using two targets for confirmation of results of the COBAS AMPLICOR Chlamydia trachomatis/Neisseria gonorrhoeae test for detection of Neisseria gonorrhoeae in clinical samples. *J Clin Microbiol.* 2005;43(5):2231-2235
Exclusion code: 4

Bohm I, Groning A, Sommer B, Muller HW, Krawczak M, Glaubitz R. A German Chlamydia trachomatis screening program employing semi-automated real-time PCR: results and perspectives. *J Clin Virol.* 2009;46 Suppl 3:S27-32
Exclusion code: 5

Bone A, Soldan K, Woodhall S, Clarke J, Gill ON. Opportunistic or population register based programmes for chlamydia screening? *BMJ.* 2012;345:e5887
Exclusion code: 7

Bongaerts M, van de Bovenkamp JHB, Morre SA, Manders MELM, Heddema ER. Evaluation of the Siemens VERSANT[REGISTERED] CT/GC DNA 1.0 assay (kPCR) for detection of Chlamydia trachomatis and Neisseria gonorrhoeae. *J Microbiol Methods.* 2011;87(2):139-142
Exclusion code: 4

Borborema-Alfaia APBd, Freitas NSdL, Astolfi Filho S, Borborema-Santos CM. Chlamydia trachomatis infection in a sample of northern Brazilian pregnant women: prevalence and prenatal importance. *Braz J Infect Dis.* 2013;17(5):545-550
Exclusion code: 5

Borel N, Kempf E, Hotzel H, et al. Direct identification of chlamydiae from clinical samples using a DNA microarray assay: a validation study. *Mol Cell Probes.* 2008;22(1):55-64
Exclusion code: 3

Appendix B4. Excluded Studies

Borges-Costa J, Matos C, Pereira F. Sexually transmitted infections in pregnant adolescents: prevalence and association with maternal and foetal morbidity. *J Eur Acad Dermatol Venereol.* 2012;26(8):972-975
Exclusion code: 5

Bott M, Bixby T, Castillo M. APTIMA Combo 2 analytical performance with C. trachomatis and N. gonorrhoeae. In: Kohl P, Jodl S, eds. *Sexually Transmitted Infections.* Bologna, Italy: Monduzzi Editore SPA; 2001:55-60
Exclusion code:Exclusion code: 7

Bowden FJ, Currie MJ, Toyne H, et al. Screening for Chlamydia trachomatis at the time of routine Pap smear in general practice: a cluster randomised controlled trial. *Med J Aust.* 2008;188(2):76-80
Exclusion code: 5

Bowden FJ, Tabrizi SN, Paterson BA, Garland SM, Fairley CK. Determination of genital human papillomavirus genotypes in women in Northern Australia using a novel, self-administered tampon technique. *Int J Gynaecol Cancer.* 1998;8(6):471-475
Exclusion code: 5

Boyadzhyan B, Yashina T, Yatabe JH, Patnaik M, Hill CS. Comparison of the APTIMA CT and GC assays with the APTIMA combo 2 assay, the Abbott LCx assay, and direct fluorescent-antibody and culture assays for detection of Chlamydia trachomatis and Neisseria gonorrhoeae. *J Clin Microbiol.* 2004;42(7):3089-3093
Exclusion code: 3

Bozicevic I, Grgic I, Zidovec-Lepej S, et al. Urine-based testing for Chlamydia trachomatis among young adults in a population-based survey in Croatia: feasibility and prevalence. *BMC Public Health.* 2011;11:230
Exclusion code: 5

Brabin L, Thomas G, Hopkins M, O'Brien K, Roberts SA. Delivery of chlamydia screening to young women requesting emergency hormonal contraception at pharmacies in Manchester, UK: a prospective study. *BMC Womens Health.* 2009;9:7
Exclusion code: 5

Bracebridge S, Bachmann MO, Ramkhelawon K, Woolnough A. Evaluation of a systematic postal screening and treatment service for genital Chlamydia trachomatis, with remote clinic access via the internet: a cross-sectional study, East of England. *Sex Transm Infect.* 2012;88(5):375-381
Exclusion code: 10

Bradley H, Satterwhite CL. Prevalence of Neisseria gonorrhoeae infections among men and women entering the National Job Training Program--United States, 2004-2009. *Sex Transm Dis.* 2012;39(1):49-54
Exclusion code: 2

Braun RA, Provost JM. Bridging the gap: using school-based health services to improve chlamydia screening among young women. *Am J Public Health.* 2010;100(9):1624-1629
Exclusion code: 4

Broad J, Cox T, Rodriguez S, et al. The impact of discontinuation of male STD screening services at a large urban county jail: Chicago, 2002-2004. *Sex Transm Dis.* 2009;36(2 Suppl):S49-52
Exclusion code: 2

Brocklehurst P. Antibiotics for gonorrhoea in pregnancy. *Cochrane database of systematic reviews (Online).* 2002(2)
Exclusion code: 2

Bromhead C, Miller A, Jones M, Whiley D. Comparison of the cobas 4800 CT/NG test with culture for detecting Neisseria gonorrhoeae in genital and nongenital specimens in a low-prevalence population in New Zealand. *J Clin Microbiol.* 2013;51(5):1505-1509
Exclusion code: 3

Brugha R, Balfe M, Conroy RM, et al. Young adults' preferred options for receiving chlamydia screening test results: a cross-sectional survey of 6085 young adults. *Int J STD AIDS.* 2011;22(11):635-639
Exclusion code: 5

Brugha R, Balfe M, Jeffares I, et al. Where do young adults want opportunistic chlamydia screening services to be located? *J Public Health (Oxf).* 2011;33(4):571-578
Exclusion code: 5

Bruine de Bruin W, Downs JS, Murray P, Fischhoff B. Can female adolescents tell whether they will test positive for Chlamydia infection? *Med Decis Making.* 2010;30(2):189-193
Exclusion code: 5

Buhrer-Skinner M, Muller R, Bialasiewicz S, et al. The check is in the mail: piloting a novel approach to Chlamydia trachomatis testing using self-collected, mailed specimen. *Sex Health.* 2009;6(2):163-169

Appendix B4. Excluded Studies

Exclusion code: 5

Buhrer-Skinner M, Muller R, Buettner PG, Gordon R, Debattista J. Improving Chlamydia trachomatis retesting rates by mailed self-collection kit. *Sex Health.* 2011;8(2):248-250
Exclusion code: 5

Buhrer-Skinner M, Muller R, Menon A, Gordon R. Novel approach to an effective community-based chlamydia screening program within the routine operation of a primary healthcare service. *Sex Health.* 2009;6(1):51-56
Exclusion code: 5

Burstein G, Jacobs A, Kissin D, Workowski K. Changes in the 2010 STD Treatment Guidelines What Adolescent Health Care Providers Should Know. 2010; The American Congress of Obstetricians and Gynecologists. http://www.acog.org/About-ACOG/ACOG-Departments/Adolescent-Health-Care/Changes-in-the-2010-STD-Treatment-Guidelines--What-Adolescent-Health-Care-Providers-Should-Know. Accessed 4 Dec, 2012
Exclusion code: 2.

Caan W. Preterm delivery in primiparous women at low risk: could epidemic chlamydia contribute to rise in preterm births? *BMJ.* 2006;332(7549):1094
Exclusion code: 7

Campbell R, Mills N, Sanford E, et al. Does population screening for Chlamydia trachomatis raise anxiety among those tested? Findings from a population based chlamydia screening study. *BMC Public Health.* 2006;6:106
Exclusion code: 2

Cano S, Fuentes M, Ballesteros J, Clavo P, Menendez B, Del Romero J. [Gonorrhea diagnoses in a center for sexually transmitted disease (STD) and their relationship with HIV and other STD, Madrid, 2005]. *Enferm Infecc Microbiol Clin.* 2009;27(6):338-341
Exclusion code: 5

Carder C, Mercey D, Benn P. Chlamydia trachomatis. *Sex Transm Infect.* 2006;82 Suppl 4:iv10-12
Exclusion code: 7

Carre H, Lindstrom R, Boman J, Janlert U, Lundqvist L, Nylander E. Asking about condom use: a key to individualized care when screening for chlamydia. *Int J STD AIDS.* 2011;22(8):436-441

Exclusion code: 5

Carvalho Gomes Hd, Velasco-Garrido M, Busse R. Screening on urogenital Chlamydia trachomatis. GMS Health Technology Assessment 2005;1. http://www.ncbi.nlm.nih.gov/pmc/articles/PMC3011323/.
Exclusion code: 6

Cassell JA, Mercer CH, Fenton KA, et al. A comparison of the population diagnosed with chlamydia in primary care with that diagnosed in sexual health clinics: implications for a national screening programme. *Public Health.* 2006;120(10):984-988
Exclusion code: 5

Castellsague X, Peeling RW, Franceschi S, et al. Chlamydia trachomatis infection in female partners of circumcised and uncircumcised adult men. *Am J Epidemiol.* 2005;162(9):907-916
Exclusion code: 4

Centers for Disease C, Prevention. Chlamydia screening among sexually active young female enrollees of health plans--United States, 1999-2001. *MMWR Morb Mortal Wkly Rep.* 2004;53(42):983-985
Exclusion code: 7

Centers for Disease C, Prevention. Chlamydia screening among sexually active young female enrollees of health plans--United States, 2000-2007.[Erratum appears in MMWR Morb Mortal Wkly Rep. 2009 Jun 12;58(22):623]. *MMWR Morb Mortal Wkly Rep.* 2009;58(14):362-365
Exclusion code: 7

Centers for Disease C, Prevention. Clinic-based testing for rectal and pharyngeal Neisseria gonorrhoeae and Chlamydia trachomatis infections by community-based organizations--five cities, United States, 2007. *MMWR Morb Mortal Wkly Rep.* 2009;58(26):716-719
Exclusion code: 7

Centers for Disease C, Prevention. CDC Grand Rounds: Chlamydia prevention: challenges and strategies for reducing disease burden and sequelae. *MMWR Morb Mortal Wkly Rep.* 2011;60(12):370-373
Exclusion code: 7

Centers for Disease Control and Prevention. Recall of LCx Neisseria gonorrhoeae Assay and Implicatons

Appendix B4. Excluded Studies

for Laboratory Testing for N. gonorrhoeae and Chlamydia trachomatis. *MMWR* 2002;51(32):709
Exclusion code: 2

Centers for Disease Control and Prevention. Male Chlamydia Screening Consultation. Atlanta, GA March 28-29 2006Exclusion code: 7

Centers for Disease Control and Prevention. Sexually Transmitted Diseases Surveillance 2010. 2011;2012(October 18). http://www.cdc.gov/std/stats10/default.htm.
Exclusion code: 2

Centers for Disease Control and Prevention. Gonorrhea - CDC Fact Sheet. 2012; Department of Health and Human Services. Atlanta, GA. Available at: http://www.cdc.gov/std/gonorrhea/STDFact-Gonorrhea.htm. Accessed October 18, 2012
Exclusion code: 2.

Centers for Disease Control and Prevention, del Rio C, Hall G, et al. Update to CDC's sexually transmitted diseases treatment guidelines, 2010: Oral cephalosporins no longer a recommended treatment for gonococcal infections. *MMWR Recomm Rep.* 2012;61(31):590-594
Exclusion code: 2

Centers for Disease Control and Prevention, Workowski KA, Berman SM. Sexually transmitted diseases treatment guidelines, 2006. *MMWR Recomm Rep.* 2006;55(RR-11):1-94
Exclusion code: 2

Centers for Disease Control and Prevention, Workowski KA, Levine WC. Sexually Transmitted Disease Treatment Guidelines--2002. *MMWR* 2002;51(RR06):1-80
Exclusion code: 2

Chacko MR, Von Sternberg K, Velasquez MM. Gonorrhea and chlamydia screening in sexually active young women: the processes of change. *J Adolesc Health.* 2004;34(5):424-427
Exclusion code: 5

Chacko MR, Wiemann CM, Smith PB. Chlamydia and gonorrhea screening in asymptomatic young women. *J Pediatr Adolesc Gynecol.* 2004;17(3):169-178
Exclusion code: 5

Chai SJ, Aumakhan B, Barnes M, et al. Internet-based screening for sexually transmitted infections to reach nonclinic populations in the community: risk

factors for infection in men. *Sex Transm Dis.* 2010;37(12):756-763
Exclusion code: 5

Chandeying V, Lamlertkittikul S, Skov S. A comparison of first-void urine, self-administered low vaginal swab, self-inserted tampon, and endocervical swab using PCR tests for the detection of infection with Chlamydia trachomatis. *Sex Health.* 2004;1(1):51-54
Exclusion code: 3

Chapin KC. Molecular tests for detection of the sexually-transmitted pathogens Neisseria gonorrhoeae and Chlamydia trachomatis. *Med Health R I.* 2006;89(6):202-204
Exclusion code: 7

Chen CS, Baeumner AJ, Durst RA. Protein G-liposomal nanovesicles as universal reagents for immunoassays. *Talanta.* 2005;67(1):205-211
Exclusion code: 4

Chen CS, Durst RA. Simultaneous detection of Escherichia coli O157:H7, Salmonella spp. and Listeria monocytogenes with an array-based immunosorbent assay using universal protein G-liposomal nanovesicles. *Talanta.* 2006;69(1):232-238
Exclusion code: 4

Chen CS, Korobkova E, Chen H, et al. A proteome chip approach reveals new DNA damage recognition activities in Escherichia coli. *Nat Methods.* 2008;5(1):69-74
Exclusion code: 4

Chen CS, Zhu H. Protein microarrays. *Biotechniques.* 2006;40(4):423, 425, 427 passim
Exclusion code: 8

Chen MY, Fairley CK, De Guingand D, et al. Screening pregnant women for chlamydia: what are the predictors of infection? *Sex Transm Infect.* 2009;85(1):31-35
Exclusion code: 5

Chen MY, Rohrsheim R, Donovan B. The differing profiles of symptomatic and asymptomatic Chlamydia trachomatis-infected men in a clinical setting. *Int J STD AIDS.* 2007;18(6):384-388
Exclusion code: 5

Chen S, Li J, van den Hoek A. Universal screening or prophylactic treatment for Chlamydia trachomatis infection among women seeking induced abortions:

Appendix B4. Excluded Studies

which strategy is more cost-effective? *Sex Transm Dis.* 2007;34(4):230-236
Exclusion code: 6

Cheney K, Wray L. Chlamydia and associated factors in an under 20s antenatal population. *Aust N Z J Obstet Gynaecol.* 2008;48(1):40-43
Exclusion code: 6

Cheng A, Kirby JE. Evaluation of the Hologic gen-probe PANTHER, APTIMA Combo 2 assay in a tertiary care teaching hospital. *Am J Clin Pathol.* 2014;141(3):397-403
Exclusion code: 4

Cheng A, Qian Q, Kirby JE. Evaluation of the Abbott RealTime CT/NG assay in comparison to the Roche Cobas Amplicor CT/NG assay. *J Clin Microbiol.* 2011;49(4):1294-1300
Exclusion code: 3

Chernesky M, Castriciano S, Jang D, Smieja M. Use of flocked swabs and a universal transport medium to enhance molecular detection of Chlamydia trachomatis and Neisseria gonorrhoeae. *J Clin Microbiol.* 2006;44(3):1084-1086
Exclusion code: 4

Chernesky M, Castriciano S, Sellors J, et al. Detection of Chlamydia trachomatis antigens in urine as an alternative to swabs and cultures. *J Infect Dis.* 1990;161(1):124-126
Exclusion code: 3

Chernesky M, Freund GG, Hook E, 3rd, Leone P, D'Ascoli P, Martens M. Detection of Chlamydia trachomatis and Neisseria gonorrhoeae infections in North American women by testing SurePath liquid-based Pap specimens in APTIMA assays. *J Clin Microbiol.* 2007;45(8):2434-2438
Exclusion code: 4

Chernesky M, Jang D, Luinstra K, et al. High analytical sensitivity and low rates of inhibition may contribute to detection of Chlamydia trachomatis in significantly more women by the APTIMA Combo 2 assay. *J Clin Microbiol.* 2006;44(2):400-405
Exclusion code: 3

Chernesky M, Jang D, Portillo E, et al. Abilities of APTIMA, AMPLICOR, and ProbeTec assays to detect Chlamydia trachomatis and Neisseria gonorrhoeae in PreservCyt ThinPrep Liquid-based Pap samples. *J Clin Microbiol.* 2007;45(8):2355-2358
Exclusion code: 4

Chernesky M, Jang D, Portillo E, et al. Comparison of three assays for detection of Chlamydia trachomatis and Neisseria gonorrhoeae in SurePath Pap samples and the role of pre- and postcytology testing. *J Clin Microbiol.* 2012;50(4):1281-1284
Exclusion code: 4

Chernesky M, Jang D, Smieja M, et al. Validation of the APTIMA Combo 2 assay for the detection of Chlamydia trachomatis and Neisseria gonorrhoeae in SurePath liquid-based pap test samples taken with different collection devices. *Sex Transm Dis.* 2009;36(9):581-583
Exclusion code: 4

Chernesky MA, Hook EW, 3rd, Martin DH, et al. Women find it easy and prefer to collect their own vaginal swabs to diagnose Chlamydia trachomatis or Neisseria gonorrhoeae infections. *Sex Transm Dis.* 2005;32(12):729-733
Exclusion code: 5

Chernesky MA, Jang DE. APTIMA transcription-mediated amplification assays for Chlamydia trachomatis and Neisseria gonorrhoeae. *Expert Rev Mol Diagn.* 2006;6(4):519-525
Exclusion code: 7

Chesson HW, Bernstein KT, Gift TL, Marcus JL, Pipkin S, Kent CK. The cost-effectiveness of screening men who have sex with men for rectal chlamydial and gonococcal infection to prevent HIV Infection. *Sex Transm Dis.* 2013;40(5):366-371
Exclusion code: 5

Chiaradonna C. The Chlamydia cascade: enhanced STD prevention strategies for adolescents. *J Pediatr Adolesc Gynecol.* 2008;21(5):233-241
Exclusion code: 7

Chidambaram JD, Melese M, Alemayehu W, et al. Mass antibiotic treatment and community protection in trachoma control programs. *Clin Infect Dis.* 2004;39(9):e95-97
Exclusion code: 3

Chojnacka K, Szczapa J, Kedzia W. [Perinatal transmission of Chlamydia trachomatis and its complication in preterm infants]. *Ginekol Pol.* 2012;83(2):116-121
Exclusion code: 8

Chow JM. Measuring the uptake and impact of Chlamydia screening programs--easier said than done. *Sex Transm Dis.* 2012;39(2):89-91
Exclusion code: 7

Appendix B4. Excluded Studies

Chrisoulidou A, Goulis DG, Iliadou PK, et al. Acute and chronic Chlamydia pneumoniae infection in pregnancy complicated with preeclampsia. *Hypertens.* 2011;30(2):164-168
Exclusion code: 5

Church DL, Amante L, Semeniuk H, Gregson DB. Selective testing of women based on age for genital Chlamydia trachomatis and Neisseria gonorrhoeae infection in a centralized regional microbiology laboratory. *Diagn Microbiol Infect Dis.* 2007;57(4):379-385
Exclusion code: 5

Clarke J, White KAJ, Turner K. Exploring short-term responses to changes in the control strategy for Chlamydia trachomatis. *Comput.* 2012;2012:803097
Exclusion code: 6

Coble BI, Nordahl-Akesson E, Vinnerberg A, Kihlstrom E. Urine-based testing for Chlamydia trachomatis using polymerase chain reaction, leucocyte esterase and urethral and cervical smears. *Scand J Clin Lab Invest.* 2006;66(4):269-277
Exclusion code: 3

Cohen DA, Nsuami M, Martin DH, Farley TA. Repeated school-based screening for sexually transmitted diseases: a feasible strategy for reaching adolescents. *Pediatrics.* 1999;104(6):1281-1285
Exclusion code: 10

Cook RL, Ostergaard L, Hillier SL, et al. Home screening for sexually transmitted diseases in high-risk young women: randomised controlled trial. *Sex Transm Infect.* 2007;83(4):286-291
Exclusion code: 3

Cornetta MdCdM, Goncalves AKdS, Bertini AM. Efficacy of cytology for the diagnosis of Chlamydia trachomatis in pregnant women. *Braz J Infect Dis.* 2006;10(5):337-340
Exclusion code: 5

Cosentino LA, Campbell T, Jett A, et al. Use of nucleic acid amplification testing for diagnosis of anorectal sexually transmitted infections. *J Clin Microbiol.* 2012;50(6):2005-2008
Exclusion code: 4

Costa A-M, Fairley CK, Garland SM, Tabrizi SN. Evaluation of self-collected urine dip swab method for detection of Chlamydia trachomatis. *Sex Health.* 2009;6(3):213-216
Exclusion code: 3

Coughlan E, Bagshaw S. Chlamydia--the problem that just won't go away. *N Z Med J.* 2005;118(1220):U1605
Exclusion code: 7

Coughlan E, Young S. Screening for pharyngeal Chlamydia trachomatis in asymptomatic men who have sex with men. *N Z Med J.* 2006;119(1232):U1948
Exclusion code: 6

Coulson R, Rao N, Freeman M. Disseminated GC infection without urogenital symptoms. *Jaapa.* 2007;20(9):29-31
Exclusion code: 6

Creighton S, Revell B, Barrow A. Concordance between nucleic acid amplification technique and culture for the diagnosis of gonorrhoea. *Int J STD AIDS.* 2009;20(5):358-359
Exclusion code: 3

Crouch SR. Opportunistic evidence: evidence-based policy in the setting of the Australian Government's chlamydia screening pilot. *Aust Health Rev.* 2012;36(1):57-60
Exclusion code: 4

Crucitti T, De Deken B, Smet H, Cuylaerts V, Abdellati S, Vuylsteke B. Evaluation of the APTIMA Combo 2 Assay using self-administered vaginal swabs for the detection of Chlamydia trachomatis and Neisseria gonorrhoeae. *Diagn Microbiol Infect Dis.* 2013;76(3):385-386
Exclusion code: 3

Culler EE, Caliendo AM, Nolte FS. Reproducibility of positive test results in the BDProbeTec ET system for detection of Chlamydia trachomatis and Neisseria gonorrhoeae. *J Clin Microbiol.* 2003;41(8):3911-3914
Exclusion code: 5

Curran G. Universal antenatal chlamydia screening by rural midwives. *Aust Nurs J.* 2012;19(7):30-32
Exclusion code: 7

Currie MJ, McNiven M, Yee T, Schiemer U, Bowden FJ. Pooling of clinical specimens prior to testing for Chlamydia trachomatis by PCR is accurate and cost saving. *J Clin Microbiol.* 2004;42(10):4866-4867
Exclusion code: 4

Currie MJ, Schmidt M, Davis BK, et al. 'Show me the money': financial incentives increase chlamydia

Appendix B4. Excluded Studies

screening rates among tertiary students: a pilot study. *Sex Health.* 2010;7(1):60-65
Exclusion code: 4

Dabrera G, Pinson D, Whiteman S. Chlamydia screening by community pharmacists: a qualitative study. *J Fam Plann Reprod Health Care.* 2011;37(1):17-21
Exclusion code: 3

Dabrera G, Pinson D, Whiteman S. Missed opportunities for chlamydia screening by community pharmacists. *Sex Health.* 2012;9(3):297
Exclusion code: 6

Dadamessi I, Eb F, Betsou F. Combined detection of Chlamydia trachomatis-specific antibodies against the 10 and 60-kDa heat shock proteins as a diagnostic tool for tubal factor infertility: Results from a case-control study in Cameroon. *FEMS Immunol Med Microbiol.* 2005;45(1):31-35
Exclusion code: 5

Dajek Z, Seliborska Z, Wiecko-Jankowska E. Assessment of direct fluorescent antibody technique in detecting Chlamydia trachomatis in sexually transmitted infections clinics. *Med Wieku Rozwoj.* 2005;9(1):111-115
Exclusion code: 4

Das S, Sabin C, Allan S. Higher vaginal pH is associated with Chlamydia trachomatis infection in women: a prospective case-controlled study. *Int J STD AIDS.* 2005;16(4):290-293
Exclusion code: 5

Das S, Sabin C, Wade A, Allan S. Sociodemography of genital co-infection with Neisseria gonorrhoeae and Chlamydia trachomatis in Coventry, UK. *Int J STD AIDS.* 2005;16(4):318-322
Exclusion code: 5

Datta SD, Sternberg M, Johnson RE, et al. Gonorrhea and Chlamydia in the United States among Persons 14 to 39 Years of Age, 1999 to 2002. *Ann Intern Med.* 2007;147(2):89-96
Exclusion code: 2

Datta SD, Torrone E, Kruszon-Moran D, et al. Chlamydia trachomatis Trends in the United States Among Persons 14 to 39 Years of Age, 1999–2008. *Sex Transm Dis.* 2012;39(2):92-96
Exclusion code: 2

Davies SC, Shepherd B, Wiig R, Kaan I. Unsupervised screening for chlamydia and

gonorrhoea in backpacker hostels in Manly, Sydney. *Sex Health.* 2013;10(2):185-187
Exclusion code: 4

De Backer E, Verhelst R, Verstraelen H, et al. Quantitative determination by real-time PCR of four vaginal Lactobacillus species, Gardnerella vaginalis and Atopobium vaginae indicates an inverse relationship between L. gasseri and L. iners. *BMC Microbiol.* 2007;7:115
Exclusion code: 3

De Martino SJ, de Barbeyrac B, Piemont Y, Barthel C, Monteil H, Jaulhac B. Detection of Chlamydia trachomatis DNA using MagNA Pure DNA extraction and Cobas Amplicor CT/NG amplification. *Clin Microbiol Infect.* 2006;12(6):576-579
Exclusion code: 4

de Silva T, Kudesia G, Joall A, Whittaker D, Davies S, Ryan C. Significance of low positive scores obtained with a method other than acceleration in the BDProbeTec-Strand displacement amplification test for detection of Neisseria gonorrhoeae. *J Clin Microbiol.* 2006;44(12):4628-4629
Exclusion code: 5

de Vries HJC, Smelov V, Ouburg S, et al. Anal lymphogranuloma venereum infection screening with IgA anti-Chlamydia trachomatis-specific major outer membrane protein serology. *Sex Transm Dis.* 2010;37(12):789-795
Exclusion code: 5

de Vries HJC, van der Bij AK, Fennema JSA, et al. Lymphogranuloma venereum proctitis in men who have sex with men is associated with anal enema use and high-risk behavior. *Sex Transm Dis.* 2008;35(2):203-208
Exclusion code: 5

de Vries R, van Bergen JEAM, de Jong-van den Berg LTW, Postma MJ, Group P-CS. Systematic screening for Chlamydia trachomatis: estimating cost-effectiveness using dynamic modeling and Dutch data. *Value Health.* 2006;9(1):1-11
Exclusion code: 5

Dean D, Turingan RS, Thomann H-U, et al. A multiplexed microfluidic PCR assay for sensitive and specific point-of-care detection of Chlamydia trachomatis. *PLoS ONE.* 2012;7(12):e51685
Exclusion code: 4

Appendix B4. Excluded Studies

Deluca GD, Marin HM, Schelover E, et al. [Chlamydia trachomatis and papillomavirus infection in women with cytohistological abnormalities in uterine cervix]. *Medicina (B Aires)*. 2006;66(4):303-306
Exclusion code: 5

den Hartog JE, Land JA, Stassen FRM, Kessels AGH, Bruggeman CA. Serological markers of persistent C. trachomatis infections in women with tubal factor subfertility. *Hum Reprod*. 2005;20(4):986-990
Exclusion code: 5

Dicker LW, Mosure DJ, Kay RS, Shelby L, Cheek JE, Region VIPP. An ongoing burden: chlamydial infections among young American Indian women. *Matern Child Health J*. 2008;12 Suppl 1:25-29
Exclusion code: 5

DiClemente RJ, Wingood GM, Rose ES, et al. Efficacy of sexually transmitted disease/human immunodeficiency virus sexual risk-reduction intervention for african american adolescent females seeking sexual health services: a randomized controlled trial. *Arch Pediatr Adolesc Med*. 2009;163(12):1112-1121
Exclusion code: 4

Dietrich W, Rath M, Stanek G, Apfalter P, Huber JC, Tempfer C. Multiple site sampling does not increase the sensitivity of Chlamydia trachomatis detection in infertility patients. *Fertil Steril*. 2010;93(1):68-71
Exclusion code: 3

Dize L, Agreda P, Quinn N, Barnes MR, Hsieh Y-H, Gaydos CA. Comparison of self-obtained penile-meatal swabs to urine for the detection of C. trachomatis, N. gonorrhoeae and T. vaginalis. *Sex Transm Infect*. 2013;89(4):305-307
Exclusion code: 4

Dodge B, Van Der Pol B, Rosenberger JG, et al. Field collection of rectal samples for sexually transmitted infection diagnostics among men who have sex with men. *Int J STD AIDS*. 2010;21(4):260-264
Exclusion code: 5

Doherty IA, Adimora AA, Schoenbach VJ, Aral SO. Correlates of gonorrhoea among African Americans in North Carolina. *Int J STD AIDS*. 2007;18(2):114-117
Exclusion code: 5

Domeika M, Oscarsson L, Hallen A, Hjelm E, Sylvan S. Mailed urine samples are not an effective screening approach for Chlamydia trachomatis case finding among young men. *J Eur Acad Dermatol Venereol*. 2007;21(6):789-794
Exclusion code: 5

Donaldson AA, Burns J, Bradshaw CP, Ellen JM, Maehr J. Screening juvenile justice-involved females for sexually transmitted infection: a pilot intervention for urban females in community supervision. *J.* 2013;19(4):258-268
Exclusion code: 6

Doseeva V, Forbes T, Wolff J, et al. Multiplex isothermal helicase-dependent amplification assay for detection of Chlamydia trachomatis and Neisseria gonorrhoeae. *Diagn Microbiol Infect Dis*. 2011;71(4):354-365
Exclusion code: 10

Downey L, Tyree PT, Lafferty WE. Preventive screening of women who use complementary and alternative medicine providers. *J Womens Health (Larchmt)*. 2009;18(8):1133-1143
Exclusion code: 4

Du P, Lemkin A, Kluhsman B, et al. The roles of social domains, behavioral risk, health care resources, and chlamydia in spatial clusters of US cervical cancer mortality: not all the clusters are the same. *Cancer Causes Control*. 2010;21(10):1669-1683
Exclusion code: 5

Durber L, Oakeshott P, Prime K, Hay P. Chlamydia screening in non-clinical settings. *Int J STD AIDS*. 2010;21(6):449-450
Exclusion code: 5

Edwards JL, Apicella MA. The molecular mechanisms used by Neisseria gonorrhoeae to initiate infection differ between men and women. *Clin Microbiol Rev*. 2004;17(4):965-981
Exclusion code: 2

Eugene JM, Hoover KW, Tao G, Kent CK. Higher yet suboptimal chlamydia testing rates at community health centers and outpatient clinics compared with physician offices. *Am J Public Health*. 2012;102(8):e26-29
Exclusion code: 5

Evans C, Das C, Kinghorn G. A retrospective study of recurrent chlamydia infection in men and women: is there a role for targeted screening for those at risk? *Int J STD AIDS*. 2009;20(3):188-192

Appendix B4. Excluded Studies

Exclusion code: 10

Fairley CK, Chen MY, Bradshaw CS, Tabrizi SN. Is it time to move to nucleic acid amplification tests screening for pharyngeal and rectal gonorrhoea in men who have sex with men to improve gonorrhoea control? *Sex Health.* 2011;8(1):9-11
Exclusion code: 7

Fairley CK, Chen S, Tabrizi S, Quinn M, Garland S. Influence of quartile of menstrual cycle on pellet volume of specimens from tampons and isolation of human papillomavirus. *J Infect Dis.* 1992;166(5):1199-1200
Exclusion code: 5

Fairley CK, Chen S, Tabrizi SN, Leeton K, Quinn MA, Garland SM. The absence of genital human papillomavirus DNA in virginal women. *Int J STD AIDS.* 1992;3(6):414-417
Exclusion code: 3

Fairley CK, Chen S, Tabrizi SN, Quinn MA, McNeil JJ, Garland SM. Tampons: a novel patient-administered method for the assessment of genital human papillomavirus infection. *J Infect Dis.* 1992;165(6):1103-1106
Exclusion code: 5

Falk L, Coble BI, Mjornberg PA, Fredlund H. Sampling for Chlamydia trachomatis infection - a comparison of vaginal, first-catch urine, combined vaginal and first-catch urine and endocervical sampling. *Int J STD AIDS.* 2010;21(4):283-287
Exclusion code: 11

Falk L, Fredlund H, Jensen JS. Symptomatic urethritis is more prevalent in men infected with Mycoplasma genitalium than with Chlamydia trachomatis. *Sex Transm Infect.* 2004;80(4):289-293
Exclusion code: 5

Fang J, Husman C, DeSilva L, Chang R, Peralta L. Evaluation of self-collected vaginal swab, first void urine, and endocervical swab specimens for the detection of Chlamydia trachomatis and Neisseria gonorrhoeae in adolescent females. *J Pediatr Adolesc Gynecol.* 2008;21(6):355-360
Exclusion code: 3

Farrell DJ. Evaluation of AMPLICOR Neisseria gonorrhoeae PCR using cppB nested PCR and 16S rRNA PCR. *J Clin Microbiol.* 1999;37(2):386-390
Exclusion code: 3

Fedorova VA, Bannikova VA, Alikberov SA, Eliseev II, Grashkin VA. [Comparative efficiency of detection of the causative agent of urogenital chlamydiasis by immunofluorescence, polymerase chain reaction, and dot immunoassay]. *Klin Lab Diagn.* 2007(7):30-35
Exclusion code: 8

Filipp E, Raczynski P, El Midaoui A, et al. Chlamydia trachomatis infection in sexually active adolescents and young women. *Med Wieku Rozwoj.* 2005;9(1):57-64
Exclusion code: 5

Finan RR, Musharrafieh U, Almawi WY. Detection of Chlamydia trachomatis and herpes simplex virus type 1 or 2 in cervical samples in human papilloma virus (HPV)-positive and HPV-negative women. *Clin Microbiol Infect.* 2006;12(9):927-930
Exclusion code: 3

Fine D, Dicker L, Mosure D, Berman S, Region XIPP. Increasing chlamydia positivity in women screened in family planning clinics: do we know why? *Sex Transm Dis.* 2008;35(1):47-52
Exclusion code: 5

Fine D, Thomas KK, Nakatsukasa-Ono W, Marrazzo J. Chlamydia positivity in women screened in family planning clinics: racial/ethnic differences and trends in the northwest U.S., 1997-2006. *Public Health Rep.* 2012;127(1):38-51
Exclusion code: 5

Fisman DN, Spain CV, Salmon ME, Goldberg M. The Philadelphia High-School STD Screening Program: key insights from dynamic transmission modeling. *Sex Transm Dis.* 2008;35(11 Suppl):S61-65
Exclusion code: 6

Forbes KM, Vaze U, Wheeler HL. Rationalization of microscopy in the detection of Neisseria gonorrhoeae in women. *Int J STD AIDS.* 2007;18(10):705-706
Exclusion code: 4

Ford CA, Pence BW, Miller WC, et al. Predicting adolescents' longitudinal risk for sexually transmitted infection: results from the National Longitudinal Study of Adolescent Health. *Arch Pediatr Adolesc Med.* 2005;159(7):657-664
Exclusion code: 5

Ford CA, Viadro CI, Miller WC. Testing for chlamydial and gonorrheal infections outside of

Appendix B4. Excluded Studies

clinic settings: a summary of the literature. *Sex Transm Dis.* 2004;31(1):38-51
Exclusion code: 4

Forni J, Miles K, Hamill M. Microscopy detection of rectal gonorrhoea in asymptomatic men. *Int J STD AIDS.* 2009;20(11):797-798
Exclusion code: 4

Forsbach-Birk V, Simnacher U, Pfrepper KI, et al. Identification and evaluation of a combination of chlamydial antigens to support the diagnosis of severe and invasive Chlamydia trachomatis infections. *Clin Microbiol Infect.* 2010;16(8):1237-1244
Exclusion code: 5

Forslin L, Kamwendo F, Bodin L, Danielsson D. [The Chlamydia infection epidemic threatens women's reproductive health. A longitudinal study points out the need of effective strategy to break the trend]. *Lakartidningen.* 2006;103(39):2848-2853
Exclusion code: 8

Foulkes HBS, Pettigrew MM, Livingston KA, Niccolai LM. Comparison of sexual partnership characteristics and associations with inconsistent condom use among a sample of adolescents and adult women diagnosed with Chlamydia trachomatis. *J Womens Health (Larchmt).* 2009;18(3):393-399
Exclusion code: 3

Fowler T, Caley M, Johal R, Brown R, Ross JDC. Previous history of gonococcal infection as a risk factor in patients presenting with gonorrhoea. *Int J STD AIDS.* 2010;21(4):277-278
Exclusion code: 5

Fowler T, Edeghere O, Inglis N, Bradshaw S. Estimating the positive predictive value of opportunistic population testing for gonorrhoea as part of the English Chlamydia Screening Programme. *Int J STD AIDS.* 2013;24(3):185-191
Exclusion code: 10

Franklin WB, Katyal M, Mahajan R, Parvez FM. Chlamydia and gonorrhea screening using urine-based nucleic acid amplification testing among males entering New York City jails: a pilot study. *J.* 2012;18(2):120-130
Exclusion code: 10

Fredlund H, Falk L, Jurstrand M, Unemo M. Molecular genetic methods for diagnosis and characterisation of Chlamydia trachomatis and Neisseria gonorrhoeae: impact on epidemiological surveillance and interventions. *Apmis.* 2004;112(11-12):771-784
Exclusion code: 7

Freeman AH, Bernstein KT, Kohn RP, Philip S, Rauch LM, Klausner JD. Evaluation of self-collected versus clinician-collected swabs for the detection of Chlamydia trachomatis and Neisseria gonorrhoeae pharyngeal infection among men who have sex with men. *Sex Transm Dis.* 2011;38(11):1036-1039
Exclusion code: 4

Friedek D, Ekiel A, Chelmicki Z, Romanik M. [HPV, Chlamydia trachomatis and genital mycoplasmas infections in women with low-grade squamous intraepithelial lesions (LSIL)]. *Ginekol Pol.* 2004;75(6):457-463
Exclusion code: 8

Friedek D, Ekiel A, Romanik M, Chelmicki Z, Chelmicki A, Martirosian G. [Chlamydia trachomatis and human papillomavirus (HPV) infections in teenage sexually active girls]. *Ginekol Pol.* 2005;76(11):879-883
Exclusion code: 8

Fruchtman Y, Greenberg D, Shany E, Melamed R, Peled N, Lifshitz M. Ophthalmia neonatorum caused by multidrug-resistant Neisseria gonorrhoeae. *Isr Med Assoc J.* 2004;6(3):180-181
Exclusion code: 3

Garland SM, Tabrizi S, Hallo J, Chen S. Assessment of Chlamydia trachomatis prevalence by PCR and LCR in women presenting for termination of pregnancy. *Sex Transm Infect.* 2000;76(3):173-176
Exclusion code: 3

Garland SM, Tabrizi SN. Diagnosis of sexually transmitted infections (STI) using self-collected non-invasive specimens. *Sex Health.* 2004;1(2):121-126
Exclusion code: 12

Garland SM, Tabrizi SN, Chen S, Byambaa C, Davaajav K. Prevalence of sexually transmitted infections (Neisseria gonorrhoeae, Chlamydia trachomatis, Trichomonas vaginalis and human papillomavirus) in female attendees of a sexually transmitted diseases clinic in Ulaanbaatar, Mongolia. *Infect Dis Obstet Gynecol.* 2001;9(3):143-146
Exclusion code: 5

Garland SM, Tabrizi SN, Fairley CK, Bowden FJ. Tampons could be used to diagnose sexually transmitted diseases. *BMJ.* 2001;322(7287):676
Exclusion code: 7

Appendix B4. Excluded Studies

Garrow SC, Smith DW, Harnett GB. The diagnosis of chlamydia, gonorrhoea, and trichomonas infections by self obtained low vaginal swabs, in remote northern Australian clinical practice. *Sex Transm Infect.* 2002;78(4):278-281
Exclusion code: 3

Garvey LJ, Roberts C, Smith A. Confirmed new HIV diagnoses in men who have sex with men after episodes of rectal gonorrhoea. *Int J STD AIDS.* 2009;20(2):144
Exclusion code: 5

Gaydos CA. Nucleic acid amplification tests for gonorrhea and chlamydia: practice and applications. *Infect Dis Clin North Am.* 2005;19(2):367-386
Exclusion code: 2

Gaydos CA, Barnes M, Aumakhan B, et al. Chlamydia trachomatis age-specific prevalence in women who used an internet-based self-screening program compared to women who were screened in family planning clinics. *Sex Transm Dis.* 2011;38(2):74-78
Exclusion code: 5

Gaydos CA, Barnes M, Dwyer K. Use of an internet program to facilitate screening for Chlamydia trachomatis. *Proc. American Society of Microbiology 105th General Meeting.* 2005
Exclusion code: 7

Gaydos CA, Cartwright CP, Colaninno P, et al. Performance of the Abbott RealTime CT/NG for detection of Chlamydia trachomatis and Neisseria gonorrhoeae. *J Clin Microbiol.* 2010;48(9):3236-3243
Exclusion code: 3

Gaydos CA, Crotchfelt KA, Shah N, et al. Evaluation of dry and wet transported intravaginal swabs in detection of Chlamydia trachomatis and Neisseria gonorrhoeae infections in female soldiers by PCR. *J Clin Microbiol.* 2002;40(3):758-761
Exclusion code: 4

Gaydos CA, Dwyer K, Barnes M, et al. Internet-based screening for Chlamydia trachomatis to reach non-clinic populations with mailed self-administered vaginal swabs.[Erratum appears in Sex Transm Dis. 2007 Aug;34(8):625]. *Sex Transm Dis.* 2006;33(7):451-457
Exclusion code: 4

Gaydos CA, Farshy C, Barnes M, et al. Can mailed swab samples be dry-shipped for the detection of

Chlamydia trachomatis, Neisseria gonorrhoeae, and Trichomonas vaginalis by nucleic acid amplification tests? *Diagn Microbiol Infect Dis.* 2012;73(1):16-20
Exclusion code: 5

Gaydos CA, McKee KT, Jr., Quinn TC, Gaydos JC. Prevalence of chlamydial and gonococcal infections among young adults.[Erratum appears in JAMA. 2004 Oct 13;292(14):1686]. *Jama.* 2004;292(7):801; author reply 801-802
Exclusion code: 7

Gaydos CA, Rizzo-Price PA, Barnes M, Dwyer K, Wood BJ, Hogan MT. The use of focus groups to design an internet-based program for chlamydia screening with self-administered vaginal swabs: what women want. *Sex Health.* 2006;3(4):209-215
Exclusion code: 5

Gaydos CA, Theodore M, Dalesio N, Wood BJ, Quinn TC. Comparison of three nucleic acid amplification tests for detection of Chlamydia trachomatis in urine specimens. *J Clin Microbiol.* 2004;42(7):3041-3045
Exclusion code: 3

Gaydos CA, Wright C, Wood BJ, Waterfield G, Hobson S, Quinn TC. Chlamydia trachomatis reinfection rates among female adolescents seeking rescreening in school-based health centers. *Sex Transm Dis.* 2008;35(3):233-237
Exclusion code: 3

Geelen TH, Rossen JW, Beerens AM, et al. Performance of cobas 4800 and m2000 real-time assays for detection of Chlamydia trachomatis and Neisseria gonorrhoeae in rectal and self-collected vaginal specimen. *Diagnostic microbiology and infectious disease.* 2013;77(2):101-105
Exclusion code: 3

Geertsen R, Friderich P, Dobec M, Emler S. Evaluation of an automated extraction method for the detection of Chlamydia trachomatis and Neisseria gonorrhoeae by Cobas Amplicor PCR from different sample materials. *Scand J Infect Dis.* 2007;39(5):405-408
Exclusion code: 4

Geisler WM. Duration of untreated, uncomplicated Chlamydia trachomatis genital infection and factors associated with chlamydia resolution: a review of human studies. *J Infect Dis.* 2010;201 Suppl 2:S104-113
Exclusion code: 7

Appendix B4. Excluded Studies

Geisler WM. Diagnosis and management of uncomplicated Chlamydia trachomatis infections in adolescents and adults: summary of evidence reviewed for the 2010 Centers for Disease Control and Prevention Sexually Transmitted Diseases Treatment Guidelines. *Clin Infect Dis.* 2011;53 Suppl 3:S92-98
Exclusion code: 7

Geisler WM, Chyu L, Kusunoki Y, Upchurch DM, Hook EW, 3rd. Health insurance coverage, health care-seeking behaviors, and genital chlamydial infection prevalence in sexually active young adults. *Sex Transm Dis.* 2006;33(6):389-396
Exclusion code: 5

Geisler WM, Tang J, Wang C, Wilson CM, Kaslow RA. Epidemiological and genetic correlates of incident Chlamydia trachomatis infection in North American adolescents. *J Infect Dis.* 2004;190(10):1723-1729
Exclusion code: 3

Geraats-Peters CWM, Brouwers M, Schneeberger PM, et al. Specific and sensitive detection of Neisseria gonorrhoeae in clinical specimens by real-time PCR. *J Clin Microbiol.* 2005;43(11):5653-5659
Exclusion code: 3

Ghanem KG, Koumans EH, Johnson RE, et al. Effect of specimen order on Chlamydia trachomatis and Neisseria gonorrhoeae test performance and adequacy of Papanicolaou smear. *J Pediatr Adolesc Gynecol.* 2006;19(1):23-30
Exclusion code: 4

Ghanem M, Radcliffe K, Allan P. The role of urethral samples in the diagnosis of gonorrhoea in women. *Int J STD AIDS.* 2004;15(1):45-47
Exclusion code: 4

Giertz G, Kallings I, Nordenvall M, Fuchs T. A prospective study of Chlamydia trachomatis infection following legal abortion. *Acta Obstet Gynecol Scand.* 1987;66(2):107-109
Exclusion code: 3

Gift TL, Gaydos CA, Kent CK, et al. The program cost and cost-effectiveness of screening men for Chlamydia to prevent pelvic inflammatory disease in women. *Sex Transm Dis.* 2008;35(11 Suppl):S66-75
Exclusion code: 6

Glass N, Nelson HD, Villemyer K. Screening for Gonorrhea: Update of the Evidence. Rockville, MD: *Quality AfHRa*;2005Exclusion code: 2

Gokral JS, Mania-Pramanik J, Meherji PK, Mali BN. Introital swab testing for Chlamydia trachomatis in a resource-poor setting: an Indian perspective. *Int J Fertil Womens Med.* 2005;50(3):140-143
Exclusion code: 3

Golden MR, Hughes JP, Cles LE, et al. Positive predictive value of Gen-Probe APTIMA Combo 2 testing for Neisseria gonorrhoeae in a population of women with low prevalence of N. gonorrhoeae infection. *Clin Infect Dis.* 2004;39(9):1387-1390
Exclusion code: 3

Goldenberg SD, Finn J, Sedudzi E, White JA, Tong CYW. Performance of the GeneXpert CT/NG assay compared to that of the Aptima AC2 assay for detection of rectal Chlamydia trachomatis and Neisseria gonorrhoeae by use of residual Aptima Samples. *J Clin Microbiol.* 2012;50(12):3867-3869
Exclusion code: 4

Golparian D, Tabrizi SN, Unemo M. Analytical specificity and sensitivity of the APTIMA Combo 2 and APTIMA GC assays for detection of commensal Neisseria species and Neisseria gonorrhoeae on the Gen-Probe Panther instrument. *Sex Transm Dis.* 2013;40(2):175-178
Exclusion code: 3

Gopal Rao G, Bacon L, Evans J, et al. Can culture confirmation of gonococcal infection be improved in female subjects found to be positive by nucleic acid amplification tests in community clinics? *Sex Transm Infect.* 2009;85(7):531-533
Exclusion code: 3

Gorbunov EF, Tsinzerling VA, Semenov NV. [Characteristics of perinatal visceral lesions caused by chlamydia trachomatis]. *Arkh Patol.* 2007;69(3):33-36
Exclusion code: 8

Gorgos L, Fine D, Marrazzo J. Chlamydia positivity in American Indian/Alaska Native women screened in family planning clinics, 1997-2004. *Sex Transm Dis.* 2008;35(8):753-757
Exclusion code: 5

Gorozpe Calvillo JI, Gomez Arzapalo E, Castaneda Vivar JJ, Santoyo Haro S, Herrera Avalos I. [Search of Chlamydia trachomatis in 159 women from private consultation]. *Ginecol Obstet Mex.* 2005;73(3):124-127
Exclusion code: 8

Appendix B4. Excluded Studies

Gottlieb SL, Berman SM, Low N. Screening and treatment to prevent sequelae in women with Chlamydia trachomatis genital infection: how much do we know? *J Infect Dis.* 2010;201 Suppl 2:S156-167
Exclusion code: 12

Gottlieb SL, Stoner BP, Zaidi AA, et al. A prospective study of the psychosocial impact of a positive Chlamydia trachomatis laboratory test. *Sex Transm Dis.* 2011;38(11):1004-1011
Exclusion code: 2

Gottlieb SL, Xu F, Brunham RC. Screening and treating Chlamydia trachomatis genital infection to prevent pelvic inflammatory disease: interpretation of findings from randomized controlled trials. *Sex Transm Dis.* 2013;40(2):97-102
Exclusion code: 12

Gotz HM, van Bergen JEAM, Veldhuijzen IK, et al. A prediction rule for selective screening of Chlamydia trachomatis infection. *Sex Transm Infect.* 2005;81(1):24-30
Exclusion code: 5

Gotz HM, van den Broek IVF, Hoebe CJPA, et al. High yield of reinfections by home-based automatic rescreening of Chlamydia positives in a large-scale register-based screening programme and determinants of repeat infections. *Sex Transm Infect.* 2013;89(1):63-69
Exclusion code: 3

Graseck AS, Secura GM, Allsworth JE, Madden T, Peipert JF. Home screening compared with clinic-based screening for sexually transmitted infections. *Obstet Gynecol.* 2010;115(4):745-752
Exclusion code: 5

Greaves A, Lonsdale S, Whinney S, Hood E, Mossop H, Olowokure B. University undergraduates' knowledge of chlamydia screening services and chlamydia infection following the introduction of a National Chlamydia Screening Programme. *Eur J Contracept Reprod Health Care.* 2009;14(1):61-68
Exclusion code: 5

Greenland KE, Op de Coul ELM, van Bergen JEAM, et al. Acceptability of the internet-based Chlamydia screening implementation in the Netherlands and insights into nonresponse. *Sex Transm Dis.* 2011;38(6):467-474
Exclusion code: 5

Griffith WF, Stuart GS, Gluck KL, Heartwell SF. Vaginal speculum lubrication and its effects on cervical cytology and microbiology. *Contraception.* 2005;72(1):60-64
Exclusion code: 4

Grover D, Prime KP, Prince MV, Ridgway G, Gilson RJC. Rectal gonorrhoea in men -- is microscopy still a useful tool? *Int J STD AIDS.* 2006;17(4):277-279
Exclusion code: 4

Gunn RA, O'Brien CJ, Lee MA, Gilchick RA. Gonorrhea screening among men who have sex with men: value of multiple anatomic site testing, San Diego, California, 1997-2003. *Sex Transm Dis.* 2008;35(10):845-848
Exclusion code: 3

Guy R, Hocking J, Low N, et al. Interventions to increase rescreening for repeat chlamydial infection. *Sex Transm Dis.* 2012;39(2):136-146
Exclusion code: 3

Guy R, Wand H, Franklin N, et al. Re-testing for chlamydia at sexual health services in Australia, 2004-08. *Sex Health.* 2011;8(2):242-247
Exclusion code: 3

Guy RJ, Ali H, Liu B, et al. Efficacy of interventions to increase the uptake of chlamydia screening in primary care: a systematic review. *BMC Infect Dis.* 2011;11:211
Exclusion code: 5

Guy RJ, Kong F, Goller J, et al. A new national Chlamydia Sentinel Surveillance System in Australia: evaluation of the first stage of implementation. *Commun Dis Intell.* 2010;34(3):319-328
Exclusion code: 5

Haasnoot A, Koedijk FDH, Op De Coul ELM, et al. Comparing two definitions of ethnicity for identifying young persons at risk for chlamydia. *Epidemiol Infect.* 2012;140(5):951-958
Exclusion code: 5

Hackett KM. Chlamydia screening. Increased efforts needed for asymptomatic women. *Adv Nurse Pract.* 2010;18(2):16
Exclusion code: 6

Hadad R, Fredlund H, Unemo M. Evaluation of the new COBAS TaqMan CT test v2.0 and impact on the proportion of new variant Chlamydia trachomatis by the introduction of diagnostics detecting new variant

Appendix B4. Excluded Studies

C trachomatis in Orebro county, Sweden. *Sex Transm Infect.* 2009;85(3):190-193
Exclusion code: 4

Haggerty CL, Gottlieb SL, Taylor BD, Low N, Xu F, Ness RB. Risk of sequelae after Chlamydia trachomatis genital infection in women. *J Infect Dis.* 2010;201 Suppl 2:S134-155
Exclusion code: 3

Hamasuna R, Hoshina S, Imai H, Jensen JS, Osada Y. Usefulness of oral wash specimens for detecting Chlamydia trachomatis from high-risk groups in Japan. *Int J Urol.* 2007;14(5):473-475
Exclusion code: 4

Hammerschlag MR. Chlamydia trachomatis and Chlamydia pneumoniae infections in children and adolescents. *Pediatr Rev.* 2004;25(2):43-51
Exclusion code: 7

Hampton T. Lymphogranuloma venereum targeted: those at risk identified; diagnostic test developed. *Jama.* 2006;295(22):2592
Exclusion code: 7

Hardwick C, White D, Osman H. An audit of the results of the Roche Amplicor gonorrhoea test on female genital samples--a cheaper and more sensitive method than culture in an urban English population. *Int J STD AIDS.* 2007;18(5):347-348
Exclusion code: 3

Harper DM, Noll WW, Belloni DR, Cole BF. Randomized clinical trial of PCR-determined human papillomavirus detection methods: self-sampling versus clinician-directed--biologic concordance and women's preferences. *Am J Obstet Gynecol.* 2002;186(3):365-373
Exclusion code: 5

Harper DM, Raymond M, Noll WW, Belloni DR, Duncan LT, Cole BF. Tampon samplings with longer cervicovaginal cell exposures are equivalent to two consecutive swabs for the detection of high-risk human papillomavirus. *Sex Transm Dis.* 2002;29(11):628-636
Exclusion code: 5

Harris DI. Implementation of chlamydia screening in a general practice setting: a 6-month pilot study. *J Fam Plann Reprod Health Care.* 2005;31(2):109-112
Exclusion code: 5

Harryman L, Scofield S, Macleod J, et al. Comparative performance of culture using swabs transported in Amies medium and the Aptima Combo 2 nucleic acid amplification test in detection of Neisseria gonorrhoeae from genital and extra-genital sites: a retrospective study. *Sex Transm Infect.* 2012;88(1):27-31
Exclusion code: 3

Haugland S, Thune T, Fosse B, Wentzel-Larsen T, Hjelmevoll SO, Myrmel H. Comparing urine samples and cervical swabs for Chlamydia testing in a female population by means of Strand Displacement Assay (SDA). *BMC Womens Health.* 2010;10:9
Exclusion code: 3

Hawthorne CM, Farber PJ, Bibbo M. Chlamydia/gonorrhea combo and HR HPV DNA testing in liquid-based pap. *Diagn Cytopathol.* 2005;33(3):177-180
Exclusion code: 5

Hay PE, Pittrof RUJ. Has the effectiveness of a single chlamydia test in preventing pelvic inflammatory disease over 12 months been overestimated? *Womens Health (Lond Engl).* 2010;6(5):627-630
Exclusion code: 7

Heijne JCM, Low N. Differential selection processes in opportunistic chlamydia screening. *Sex Transm Infect.* 2011;87(6):454-455
Exclusion code: 7

Heijne JCM, Tao G, Kent CK, Low N. Uptake of regular chlamydia testing by U.S. women: a longitudinal study. *Am J Prev Med.* 2010;39(3):243-250
Exclusion code: 5

Hennrikus E, Oberto D, Linder JM, Rempel JML, Hennrikus N. Sports preparticipation examination to screen college athletes for Chlamydia trachomatis. *Med Sci Sports Exerc.* 2010;42(4):683-688
Exclusion code: 10

Herring A, Ballard R, Mabey D, Peeling RW, Initiative WTSTDD. Evaluation of rapid diagnostic tests: chlamydia and gonorrhoea. *Nature Reviews Microbiology.* 2006;4(12 Suppl):S41-48
Exclusion code: 7

Hince D, Brett T, Mak D, Bulsara M, Moorhead R, Arnold-Reed D. Opportunistic screening for chlamydia in young men. *Aust Fam Physician.* 2009;38(9):734-737
Exclusion code: 10

Appendix B4. Excluded Studies

Hislop J, Quayyum Z, Flett G, Boachie C, Fraser C, Mowatt G. Systematic review of the clinical effectiveness and cost-effectiveness of rapid point-of-care tests for the detection of genital chlamydia infection in women and men. *Health Technol Assess.* 2010;14(29):1-97, iii-iv
Exclusion code: 4

Hjelmevoll SO, Olsen ME, Sollid JUE, et al. Clinical validation of a real-time polymerase chain reaction detection of Neisseria gonorrheae porA pseudogene versus culture techniques. *Sex Transm Dis.* 2008;35(5):517-520
Exclusion code: 3

Hjelmevoll SO, Olsen ME, Sollid JUE, Haaheim H, Unemo M, Skogen V. A fast real-time polymerase chain reaction method for sensitive and specific detection of the Neisseria gonorrhoeae porA pseudogene. *J Mol Diagn.* 2006;8(5):574-581
Exclusion code: 3

Ho MK, Lo JYC, Lo ACT, Cheng FK, Chan FK. Evaluation of replacing the existing diagnostic strategy for Neisseria gonorrhoeae and Chlamydia trachomatis infections with sole molecular testing of urine specimens in a sexually transmitted infection clinic setting. *Sex Transm Infect.* 2009;85(5):322-325
Exclusion code: 3

Hocking J, Fairley CK. Do the characteristics of sexual health centre clients predict chlamydia infection sufficiently strongly to allow selective screening? *Sex Health.* 2005;2(3):185-192
Exclusion code: 5

Hodgins S, Peeling RW, Dery S, et al. The value of mass screening for chlamydia control in high prevalence communities. *Sex Transm Infect.* 2002;78 Suppl 1:i64-68
Exclusion code: 3

Hogan AH, Howell-Jones RS, Pottinger E, Wallace LM, McNulty CA. "...they should be offering it": a qualitative study to investigate young peoples' attitudes towards chlamydia screening in GP surgeries. *BMC Public Health.* 2010;10:616
Exclusion code: 4

Holden AEC, Shain RN, Miller WB, et al. The influence of depression on sexual risk reduction and STD infection in a controlled, randomized intervention trial. *Sex Transm Dis.* 2008;35(10):898-904
Exclusion code: 3

Holland D. Chlamydia screening: making a case for including men. *Nurs Times.* 2006;102(13):44-46
Exclusion code: 7

Hollegaard S, Vogel I, Thorsen P, Jensen IP, Mordhorst C-H, Jeune B. Chlamydia trachomatis C-complex serovars are a risk factor for preterm birth. *In Vivo.* 2007;21(1):107-112
Exclusion code: 3

Hood EE, Nerhood RC. The utility of screening for chlamydia at 34-36 weeks gestation. *W V Med J.* 2010;106(6):10-11
Exclusion code: 5

Hook EW, 3rd, Ching SF, Stephens J, Hardy KF, Smith KR, Lee HH. Diagnosis of Neisseria gonorrhoeae infections in women by using the ligase chain reaction on patient-obtained vaginal swabs. *J Clin Microbiol.* 1997;35(8):2129-2132
Exclusion code: 3

Hook EW, 3rd, Smith K, Mullen C, et al. Diagnosis of genitourinary Chlamydia trachomatis infections by using the ligase chain reaction on patient-obtained vaginal swabs. *J Clin Microbiol.* 1997;35(8):2133-2135
Exclusion code: 3

Hopkins MJ, Ashton LJ, Alloba F, Alawattegama A, Hart IJ. Validation of a laboratory-developed real-time PCR protocol for detection of Chlamydia trachomatis and Neisseria gonorrhoeae in urine. *Sex Transm Infect.* 2010;86(3):207-211
Exclusion code: 3

Hopkins MJ, Smith G, Hart IJ, Alloba F. Screening tests for Chlamydia trachomatis or Neisseria gonorrhoeae using the cobas 4800 PCR system do not require a second test to confirm: an audit of patients issued with equivocal results at a sexual health clinic in the Northwest of England, U.K. *Sex Transm Infect.* 2012;88(7):495-497
Exclusion code: 5

Hopwood J, Mallinson H, Hodgson E, Hull L. Liquid based cytology: examination of its potential in a chlamydia screening programme. *Sex Transm Infect.* 2004;80(5):371-373
Exclusion code: 4

Horner P, Skidmore S, Herring A, et al. Enhanced enzyme immunoassay with negative-gray-zone testing compared to a single nucleic Acid amplification technique for community-based

Appendix B4. Excluded Studies

chlamydial screening of men. *J Clin Microbiol.* 2005;43(5):2065-2069
Exclusion code: 3

Horner PJ. Should we still be testing for asymptomatic non-specific urethritis in departments of genitourinary medicine? *Int J STD AIDS.* 2005;16(4):273-277
Exclusion code: 7

Hu D, Hook EW, 3rd, Goldie SJ. The impact of natural history parameters on the cost-effectiveness of Chlamydia trachomatis screening strategies. *Sex Transm Dis.* 2006;33(7):428-436
Exclusion code: 6

Huppert JS, Biro F, Lan D, Mortensen JE, Reed J, Slap GB. Urinary symptoms in adolescent females: STI or UTI? *J Adolesc Health.* 2007;40(5):418-424
Exclusion code: 3

Huppert JS, Mortensen JE, Reed JL, Kahn JA, Rich KD, Hobbs MM. Mycoplasma genitalium detected by transcription-mediated amplification is associated with Chlamydia trachomatis in adolescent women. *Sex Transm Dis.* 2008;35(3):250-254
Exclusion code: 5

Hurly DS, Buhrer-Skinner M, Badman SG, et al. Field evaluation of the CRT and ACON chlamydia point-of-care tests in a tropical, low-resource setting. *Sex Transm Infect.* 2014;90(3):179-184
Exclusion code: 4

Hwang LY, Tebb KP, Shafer M-AB, Pantell RH. Examination of the treatment and follow-up care for adolescents who test positive for Chlamydia trachomatis infection. *Arch Pediatr Adolesc Med.* 2005;159(12):1162-1166
Exclusion code: 3

Imai H, Shinohara H, Nakao H, Tsukino H, Hamasuna R, Katoh T. Prevalence and risk factors of asymptomatic chlamydial infection among students in Japan. *Int J STD AIDS.* 2004;15(6):408-414
Exclusion code: 5

Irvin CB, Nowak B, Moore M, Flynn K, Vretta C. Emergency department Chlamydia screening through partnership with the public health department. *Acad Emerg Med.* 2009;16(11):1217-1220
Exclusion code: 10

Irwig L, Tosteson ANA, Gatsonis C, et al. Guidelines for Meta-analyses Evaluating Diagnostic Tests. *Ann Intern Med.* 1994;120(8):667-676

Exclusion code: 2

Iur'ev SI, Krotov SA, Degteva SS, et al. [Perinatal aspects of serological diagnosis in urogenital chlamydiosis]. *Klin Lab Diagn.* 2005(3).20-23
Exclusion code: 8

Jalal H, Al-Suwaine A, Stephen H, Carne C, Sonnex C. Comparative performance of the Roche COBAS Amplicor assay and an in-house real-time PCR assay for diagnosis of Chlamydia trachomatis infection. *J Med Microbiol.* 2007;56(Pt 3):320-322
Exclusion code: 4

Jalal H, Stephen H, Al-Suwaine A, Sonnex C, Carne C. The superiority of polymerase chain reaction over an amplified enzyme immunoassay for the detection of genital chlamydial infections. *Sex Transm Infect.* 2006;82(1):37-40
Exclusion code: 3

Jalkh AP, Miranda AE, Hurtado-Guerreiro JC, et al. Chlamydia trachomatis in human immunodeficiency virus-infected men treated at a referral hospital for sexually transmitted diseases in the Amazonas, Brazil. *Braz J Infect Dis.* 2014;18(2):158-163
Exclusion code: 3

Jamil MS, Hocking JS, Bauer HM, et al. Home-based chlamydia and gonorrhoea screening: a systematic review of strategies and outcomes. *BMC Public Health.* 2013;13:189
Exclusion code: 5

Jaton K, Bille J, Greub G. A novel real-time PCR to detect Chlamydia trachomatis in first-void urine or genital swabs. *J Med Microbiol.* 2006;55(Pt 12):1667-1674
Exclusion code: 4

Jenkins WD, Kovach R, Wold BJ, Zahnd WE. Using patient-provided information to refine sexually transmitted infection screening criteria among women presenting in the emergency department. *Sex Transm Dis.* 2012;39(12):965-967
Exclusion code: 5

Jenkins WD, Kruse J. Chlamydia screening: how we can better serve patients. *J.* 2010;59(2):E2
Exclusion code: 7

Jenkins WD, Nessa LL, Clark T. Cross-sectional study of pharyngeal and genital chlamydia and gonorrhoea infections in emergency department patients. *Sex Transm Infect.* 2014;90(3):246-249
Exclusion code: 5

Appendix B4. Excluded Studies

Jenkins WD, Weis R, Campbell P, Barnes M, Barnes P, Gaydos C. Comparative effectiveness of two self-collected sample kit distribution systems for chlamydia screening on a university campus. *Sex Transm Infect.* 2012;88(5):363-367
Exclusion code: 4

Jenkins WD, Zahnd W, Kovach R, Kissinger P. Chlamydia and gonorrhea screening in United States emergency departments. *J Emerg Med.* 2013;44(2):558-567
Exclusion code: 2

Jensen JS, Bjornelius E, Dohn B, Lidbrink P. Comparison of first void urine and urogenital swab specimens for detection of Mycoplasma genitalium and Chlamydia trachomatis by polymerase chain reaction in patients attending a sexually transmitted disease clinic. *Sex Transm Dis.* 2004;31(8):499-507
Exclusion code: 3

Jespersen DJ, Flatten KS, Jones MF, Smith TF. Prospective comparison of cell cultures and nucleic acid amplification tests for laboratory diagnosis of Chlamydia trachomatis Infections. *J Clin Microbiol.* 2005;43(10):5324-5326
Exclusion code: 3

Joesoef MR, Mosure DJ. Prevalence of Chlamydia in young men in the United States from newly implemented universal screening in a national job training program. *Sex Transm Dis.* 2006;33(10):636-639
Exclusion code: 5

Joesoef MR, Weinstock HS, Johnson RE. Factors associated with recurrent chlamydial infection and failure to return for retesting in young women entering national job training program, 1998--2005. *Sex Transm Dis.* 2008;35(4):368-371
Exclusion code: 3

Joffe A, Rietmeijer CA, Chung S-E, et al. Screening asymptomatic adolescent men for Chlamydia trachomatis in school-based health centers using urine-based nucleic acid amplification tests. *Sex Transm Dis.* 2008;35(11 Suppl):S19-23
Exclusion code: 5

Johnson CC, Jones EH, Goldberg M, Asbel LE, Salmon ME, Waller CL. Screening for Chlamydia trachomatis and Neisseria gonorrhoeae among adolescents in Family Court, Philadelphia, Pennsylvania. *Sex Transm Dis.* 2008;35(11 Suppl):S24-27
Exclusion code: 10

Johnson RE, Green TA, Schachter J, et al. Evaluation of nucleic acid amplification tests as reference tests for Chlamydia trachomatis infections in asymptomatic men. *J Clin Microbiol.* 2000;38(12):4382-4386
Exclusion code: 10

Johnson SA, Simms I, Sheringham J, et al. The implementation of chlamydia screening: a cross-sectional study in the south east of England. *Sex Transm Infect.* 2010;86(3):217-221
Exclusion code: 6

Jones HE, Altini L, de Kock A, Young T, van de Wijgert JH. Home-based versus clinic-based self-sampling and testing for sexually transmitted infections in Gugulethu, South Africa: randomised controlled trial. *Sex Transm Infect.* 2007;83(7):552-557
Exclusion code: 5

Jones K, Baldwin KA, Lewis PR. The potential influence of a social media intervention on risky sexual behavior and Chlamydia incidence. *J Community Health Nurs.* 2012;29(2):106-120
Exclusion code: 4

Jordan NN, Clemmons NS, Gaydos JC, Lee H-CS, Yi SH, Klein TA. Chlamydia trachomatis screening initiative among U.S. Army soldiers assigned to Korea. *Msmr.* 2013;20(2):15-16
Exclusion code: 5

Joyee AG, Thyagarajan SP, Reddy EV, Venkatesan C, Ganapathy M. Genital chlamydial infection in STD patients: its relation to HIV infection. *Indian J.* 2005;23(1):37-40
Exclusion code: 3

Jumping-Eagle S, Sheeder J, Kelly LS, Stevens-Simon C. Feasibility and utility of screening adolescent mothers for Chlamydia at their children's health care visits. *Matern Child Health J.* 2007;11(6):586-594
Exclusion code: 10

Kadzhaia D, Merabishvili N. Prevalence and risk factors for Chlamydia trachomatis infection in pregnant women. *Georgian Med.* 2005(129):33-36
Exclusion code: 5

Kalwij S, Macintosh M, Baraitser P. Screening and treatment of Chlamydia trachomatis infections. *BMJ.* 2010;340:c1915
Exclusion code: 7

Appendix B4. Excluded Studies

Kalwij SA. Opportunistic chlamydia screening in a general practice consultation. *BMJ.* 2011;343:d5108
Exclusion code: 7

Kangas I, Andersen B, Olesen F, Moller JK, Ostergaard L. Psychosocial impact of Chlamydia trachomatis testing in general practice. *Br J Gen Pract.* 2006;56(529):587-593
Exclusion code: 3

Kanno MB, Nguyen RHN, Lee EM, Zenilman JM, Erbelding EJ. The prevalence of abnormal cervical cytology in a sexually transmitted diseases clinic. *Int J STD AIDS.* 2005;16(8):549-552
Exclusion code: 3

Kapala J, Biers K, Cox M, et al. Aptima Combo 2 testing detected additional cases of Neisseria gonorrhoeae infection in men and women in community settings. *J Clin Microbiol.* 2011;49(5):1970-1971
Exclusion code: 3

Karinen L, Pouta A, Bloigu A, et al. Serum C-reactive protein and Chlamydia trachomatis antibodies in preterm delivery. *Obstet Gynecol.* 2005;106(1):73-80
Exclusion code: 5

Karowicz-Biliniska A, Kus E, Kazimiera W, et al. [Chlamydia trachomatis infection and bacterial analysis in pregnant women in II and III trimester of pregnancy]. *Ginekol Pol.* 2007;78(10):787-791
Exclusion code: 8

Kasowitz AR, McCusker M, Coury-Doniger P, et al. Stage of change behavioral assessment tool fails to predict the prevalence of chlamydia in an urban adolescent health clinic. *J Pediatr Adolesc Gynecol.* 2006;19(4):277-283
Exclusion code: 5

Keegan H, Malkin A, Griffin M, Ryan F, Lambkin H. Validation of a multiplex PCR assay for the simultaneous detection of human papillomavirus and Chlamydia trachomatis in cervical PreservCyt samples. *Clin Chem.* 2005;51(7):1301-1302
Exclusion code: 3

Kehl SC, Georgakas K, Swain GR, et al. Evaluation of the abbott LCx assay for detection of Neisseria gonorrhoeae in endocervical swab specimens from females. *J Clin Microbiol.* 1998;36(12):3549-3551
Exclusion code: 3

Keltz MD, Sauerbrun-Cutler M-T, Durante MS, Moshier E, Stein DE, Gonzales E. Positive Chlamydia trachomatis serology result in women seeking care for infertility is a negative prognosticator for intrauterine pregnancy. *Sex Transm Dis.* 2013;40(11):842-845
Exclusion code: 5

Kent CK, Chaw JK, Wong W, et al. Prevalence of rectal, urethral, and pharyngeal chlamydia and gonorrhea detected in 2 clinical settings among men who have sex with men: San Francisco, California, 2003. *Clin Infect Dis.* 2005;41(1):67-74
Exclusion code: 3

Kerndt PR, Ferrero DV, Aynalem G, et al. First report of performance of the Versant CT/GC DNA 1.0 assay (kPCR) for detection of Chlamydia trachomatis and Neisseria gonorrhoeae. *J Clin Microbiol.* 2011;49(4):1347-1353
Exclusion code: 4

Khan A, Hussain R, Schofield M. Correlates of sexually transmitted infections in young Australian women. *Int J STD AIDS.* 2005;16(7):482-487
Exclusion code: 5

Khan ER, Hossain MA, Paul SK, et al. Comparison between ICT and PCR for diagnosis of Chlamydia trachomatis. *Mymensingh Med J.* 2012;21(2):190-194
Exclusion code: 4

Khandhadia S, Foster S, Cree A, et al. Chlamydia infection status, genotype, and age-related macular degeneration. *Mol Vis.* 2012;18:29-37
Exclusion code: 5

Khryanin AA, Reshetnikov OV, Vlaspolder F. Comparison of APTIMA COMBO 2 assay with polymerase chain reaction Roche assay for detection of Chlamydia trachomatis in endocervical swabs. *Int J STD AIDS.* 2007;18(12):871-872
Exclusion code: 3

Killick V, Kell P, Plumb H, Hurd N, Turner P. Screening for Neisseria gonorrhoeae using the BD ProbeTec nucleic acid amplification test in a low prevalence genitourinary medicine clinic. *Int J STD AIDS.* 2012;23(6):e1-3
Exclusion code: 3

Kimmitt PT, Tabrizi SN, Crosatti M, et al. Pilot study of the utility and acceptability of tampon sampling for the diagnosis of Neisseria gonorrhoeae and Chlamydia trachomatis infections by duplex realtime

Appendix B4. Excluded Studies

polymerase chain reaction in United Kingdom sex workers. *Int J STD AIDS.* 2010;21(4):279-282
Exclusion code: 5

Kirk E, Bora S, Van Calster B, et al. Chlamydia trachomatis infection in patients attending an Early Pregnancy Unit: prevalence, symptoms, pregnancy location and viability. *Acta Obstet Gynecol Scand.* 2008;87(6):601-607
Exclusion code: 5

Klovstad H, Natas O, Tverdal A, Aavitsland P. Systematic screening with information and home sampling for genital Chlamydia trachomatis infections in young men and women in Norway: a randomized controlled trial. *BMC Infect Dis.* 2013;13:30
Exclusion code: 5

Knesel BW, Dry JC, Wald-Scott C, Aftab A. Preliminary evaluation of a cervical self-sampling device with liquid-based cytology and multiparameter molecular testing.[Erratum appears in J Reprod Med. 2005 May;50(5):376 Note: Aftoh, Asma [corrected to Aftab, Asma]]. *J Reprod Med.* 2005;50(4):256-260
Exclusion code: 5

Knox J, Tabrizi SN, Miller P, et al. Evaluation of self-collected samples in contrast to practitioner-collected samples for detection of Chlamydia trachomatis, Neisseria gonorrhoeae, and Trichomonas vaginalis by polymerase chain reaction among women living in remote areas. *Sex Transm Dis.* 2002;29(11):647-654
Exclusion code: 3

Koffi SK, Faye-Kette H, Kacou-N'douba A, Kouassi-M'bengue A, Dosso M. [Evaluation of first void urine in the detection of Neisseria gonorrhoeae in patients less symptomatic in Abidjan (Cote d'Ivoire)]. *Med Trop (Mars).* 2009;69(3):275-277
Exclusion code: 8

Korenromp EL, White RG, Orroth KK, et al. Determinants of the impact of sexually transmitted infection treatment on prevention of HIV infection: a synthesis of evidence from the Mwanza, Rakai, and Masaka intervention trials. *J Infect Dis.* 2005;191 Suppl 1:S168-178
Exclusion code: 4

Koumans EH, Black CM, Markowitz LE, et al. Comparison of methods for detection of Chlamydia trachomatis and Neisseria gonorrhoeae using commercially available nucleic acid amplification tests and a liquid pap smear medium. *J Clin Microbiol.* 2003;41(4):1507-1511
Exclusion code: 3

Koumans EHA, Rosen J, van Dyke MK, et al. Prevention of mother-to-child transmission of infections during pregnancy: implementation of recommended interventions, United States, 2003-2004. *Am J Obstet Gynecol.* 2012;206(2):158.e151-158.e111
Exclusion code: 5

Kouyoumdjian FG, Leto D, John S, Henein H, Bondy S. A systematic review and meta-analysis of the prevalence of chlamydia, gonorrhoea and syphilis in incarcerated persons. *Int J STD AIDS.* 2012;23(4):248-254
Exclusion code: 5

Krech T, Castriciano S, Jang D, Smieja M, Enders G, Chernesky M. Detection of high risk HPV and Chlamydia trachomatis in vaginal and cervical samples collected with flocked nylon and wrapped rayon dual swabs transported in dry tubes. *J Virol Methods.* 2009;162(1-2):291-293
Exclusion code: 4

Kretzschmar M, Satterwhite C, Leichliter J, Berman S. Effects of screening and partner notification on Chlamydia positivity in the United States: a modeling study. *Sex Transm Dis.* 2012;39(5):325-331
Exclusion code: 6

Kretzschmar M, Turner KME, Barton PM, Edmunds WJ, Low N. Predicting the population impact of chlamydia screening programmes: comparative mathematical modelling study. *Sex Transm Infect.* 2009;85(5):359-366
Exclusion code: 6

Kwan B, Ryder N, Knight V, et al. Sensitivity of 20-minute voiding intervals in men testing for Chlamydia trachomatis. *Sex Transm Dis.* 2012;39(5):405-406
Exclusion code: 5

La Montagne DS, Patrick LE, Fine DN, Marrazzo JM, Region XIPP. Re-evaluating selective screening criteria for chlamydial infection among women in the U S Pacific Northwest. *Sex Transm Dis.* 2004;31(5):283-289
Exclusion code: 3

LaMontagne DS, Fenton KA, Randall S, Anderson S, Carter P. Establishing the National Chlamydia Screening Programme in England: results from the

Appendix B4. Excluded Studies

first full year of screening. *Sex Transm Infect.* 2004;80(5):335-341
Exclusion code: 10

Langille DB, Proudfoot K, Rigby J, Aquino-Russell C, Strang R, Forward K. A pilot project for chlamydia screening in adolescent females using self-testing: characteristics of participants and non-participants. *Can J Public Health.* 2008;99(2):117-120
Exclusion code: 5

Lardenoije CMJG, Land JA. [Chlamydia antibody testing for tubal factor subfertility]. *Ned Tijdschr Geneeskd.* 2007;151(36):1981-1985
Exclusion code: 8

Lavelle SJ, Jones KE, Mallinson H, Webb AMC. Finding, confirming, and managing gonorrhoea in a population screened for chlamydia using the Gen-Probe Aptima Combo2 assay. *Sex Transm Infect.* 2006;82(3):221-224
Exclusion code: 3

Lawless S. Sustaining chlamydia screening is difficult. *J Prim Health Care.* 2010;2(4):347
Exclusion code: 7

Lawton B, Rose S, Bromhead C, Brown S, MacDonald J, Shepherd J. Rates of Chlamydia trachomatis testing and chlamydial infection in pregnant women. *N Z Med J.* 2004;117(1194):U889
Exclusion code: 5

Lawton BA, Rose SB, Elley CR, Bromhead C, MacDonald EJ, Baker MG. Increasing the uptake of opportunistic chlamydia screening: a pilot study in general practice. *J Prim Health Care.* 2010;2(3):199-207
Exclusion code: 5

Lawung R, Cherdtrakulkiat R, Charoenwatanachokchai A, Nabu S, Suksaluk W, Prachayasittikul V. One-step PCR for the identification of multiple antimicrobial resistance in Neisseria gonorrhoeae. *J Microbiol Methods.* 2009;77(3):323-325
Exclusion code: 5

Le Roy C, Le Hen I, Clerc M, et al. The first performance report for the Bio-Rad Dx CT/NG/MG assay for simultaneous detection of Chlamydia trachomatis, Neisseria gonorrhoeae and Mycoplasma genitalium in urogenital samples. *J Microbiol Methods.* 2012;89(3):193-197
Exclusion code: 3

Lee JY, Lensing SY, Schwebke JR. Retention of clinical trial participants in a study of nongonococcal urethritis (NGU), a sexually transmitted infection in men. *Contemp Clin Trials.* 2012;33(4):606-610
Exclusion code: 5

Lee SH, Vigliotti VS, Pappu S. DNA sequencing validation of Chlamydia trachomatis and Neisseria gonorrhoeae nucleic acid tests. *Am J Clin Pathol.* 2008;129(6):852-859
Exclusion code: 4

Lee SH, Vigliotti VS, Pappu S. Molecular tests for human papillomavirus (HPV), Chlamydia trachomatis and Neisseria gonorrhoeae in liquid-based cytology specimen. *BMC Womens Health.* 2009;9:8
Exclusion code: 5

Lee S-J, Park DC, Lee DS, Choe H-S, Cho Y-H. Evaluation of Seeplex STD6 ACE Detection kit for the diagnosis of six bacterial sexually transmitted infections. *J Infect Chemother.* 2012;18(4):494-500
Exclusion code: 3

Lee SR, Chung JM, Kim YG. Rapid one step detection of pathogenic bacteria in urine with sexually transmitted disease (STD) and prostatitis patient by multiplex PCR assay (mPCR). *J.* 2007;45(5):453-459
Exclusion code: 4

Lee V, Tobin JM, Foley E. Relationship of cervical ectopy to chlamydia infection in young women. *J Fam Plann Reprod Health Care.* 2006;32(2):104-106
Exclusion code: 5

Lee YM, Samaranayake A, Fairley CK, et al. Pelvic examination leads to changed clinical management in very few women diagnosed with asymptomatic chlamydia infection. *Sex Health.* 2010;7(4):498-499
Exclusion code: 10

Lehtinen M, Ault KA, Lyytikainen E, et al. Chlamydia trachomatis infection and risk of cervical intraepithelial neoplasia. *Sex Transm Infect.* 2011;87(5):372-376
Exclusion code: 5

Levett PN, Brandt K, Olenius K, Brown C, Montgomery K, Horsman GB. Evaluation of three automated nucleic acid amplification systems for detection of Chlamydia trachomatis and Neisseria gonorrhoeae in first-void urine specimens. *J Clin Microbiol.* 2008;46(6):2109-2111
Exclusion code: 3

Appendix B4. Excluded Studies

Levi AW, Beckman D, Hui P, Schofield K, Harigopal M, Chhieng DC. Comparing two methods of detection for Chlamydia trachomatis in liquid-based Papanicolaou tests. *Am J Clin Pathol.* 2012;138(2):236-240
Exclusion code: 4

Levy V, Blackmore CS, Klausner JD. Self-collection of specimens for nucleic acid-based diagnosis of pharyngeal, cervicovaginal, urethral, and rectal Neisseria gonorrhoeae and Chlamydia trachomatis infections. *Methods Mol Biol.* 2012;903:407-418
Exclusion code: 7

Li J-H, Yin Y-P, Zheng H-P, et al. A high-resolution melting analysis for genotyping urogenital Chlamydia trachomatis. *Diagn Microbiol Infect Dis.* 2010;68(4):366-374
Exclusion code: 4

Lin KW, Ramsey L. Screening for chlamydial infection. *Am Fam Physician.* 2008;78(12):1349-1350
Exclusion code: 7

Lindan C, Mathur M, Kumta S, et al. Utility of pooled urine specimens for detection of Chlamydia trachomatis and Neisseria gonorrhoeae in men attending public sexually transmitted infection clinics in Mumbai, India, by PCR. *J Clin Microbiol.* 2005;43(4):1674-1677
Exclusion code: 4

Lister NA, Tabrizi SN, Fairley CK, Garland S. Validation of roche COBAS Amplicor assay for detection of Chlamydia trachomatis in rectal and pharyngeal specimens by an omp1 PCR assay. *J Clin Microbiol.* 2004;42(1):239-241
Exclusion code: 4

Lloyd TDR, Malin G, Pugsley H, et al. Women presenting with lower abdominal pain: a missed opportunity for chlamydia screening? *Surg.* 2006;4(1):15-19
Exclusion code: 6

Lofy KH, Hofmann J, Mosure DJ, Fine DN, Marrazzo JM. Chlamydial infections among female adolescents screened in juvenile detention centers in Washington State, 1998-2002. *Sex Transm Dis.* 2006;33(2):63-67
Exclusion code: 5

Logan S, Browne J, McKenzie H, Templeton A, Bhattacharya S. Evaluation of endocervical, first-void urine and self-administered vulval swabs for the detection of Chlamydia trachomatis in a miscarriage population.[Erratum appears in BJOG. 2005 Apr;112(4):528]. *Bjog.* 2005;112(1):103-106
Exclusion code: 3

Lorimer K. Pilot qualitative analysis of the psychosocial factors which drive young people to decline chlamydia testing in the UK: implications for health promotion and screening. *Int J STD AIDS.* 2010;21(5):379
Exclusion code: 7

Lorimer K, Hart GJ. Knowledge of Chlamydia trachomatis among men and women approached to participate in community-based screening, Scotland, UK. *BMC Public Health.* 2010;10:794
Exclusion code: 5

Low N. Current status of Chlamydia screening in Europe. *Euro Surveill.* 2004;8(41)
Exclusion code: 7

Low N. Evaluating novel interventions for chlamydia screening. *Sex Transm Infect.* 2006;82(2):97-98
Exclusion code: 7

Low N, Bender N, Nartey L, Shang A, Stephenson JM. Effectiveness of chlamydia screening: systematic review. *Int J Epidemiol.* 2009;38(2):435-448
Exclusion code: 12

Low N, Egger M, Sterne JAC, et al. Incidence of severe reproductive tract complications associated with diagnosed genital chlamydial infection: the Uppsala Women's Cohort Study. *Sex Transm Infect.* 2006;82(3):212-218
Exclusion code: 3

Low N, Harbord RM, Egger M, Sterne JA, Herrmann B. Screening for chlamydia. *Lancet.* 2005;365(9470):1539
Exclusion code: 5

Low N, McCarthy A, Macleod J, et al. Epidemiological, social, diagnostic and economic evaluation of population screening for genital chlamydial infection. *Health Technol Assess.* 2007;11(8):iii-iv, ix-xii, 1-165
Exclusion code: 3

Low N, McCarthy A, Macleod J, et al. The chlamydia screening studies: rationale and design. *Sex Transm Infect.* 2004;80(5):342-348
Exclusion code: 2

Lowe P, O'Loughlin P, Evans K, White M, Bartley PB, Vohra R. Comparison of the Gen-Probe

Appendix B4. Excluded Studies

APTIMA Combo 2 assay to the AMPLICOR CT/NG assay for detection of Chlamydia trachomatis and Neisseria gonorrhoeae in urine samples from Australian men and women. *J Clin Microbiol.* 2006;44(7):2619-2621
Exclusion code: 3

Luijt DS, Bos PAJ, van Zwet AA, van Voorst Vader PC, Schirm J. Comparison of COBAS AMPLICOR Neisseria gonorrhoeae PCR, including confirmation with N. gonorrhoeae-specific 16S rRNA PCR, with traditional culture. *J Clin Microbiol.* 2005;43(3):1445-1447
Exclusion code: 3

Lum G, Garland SM, Tabrizi S, et al. Supplemental testing is still required in australia for samples positive for Neisseria gonorrhoeae by nucleic acid detection tests. *J Clin Microbiol.* 2006;44(11):4292-4294; author reply 4293-4294
Exclusion code: 7

Luostarinen T, Lehtinen M, Bjorge T, et al. Joint effects of different human papillomaviruses and Chlamydia trachomatis infections on risk of squamous cell carcinoma of the cervix uteri. *Eur J Cancer.* 2004;40(7):1058-1065
Exclusion code: 4

MacDonald N, Mailman T, Desai S. Gonococcal infections in newborns and in adolescents. *Adv Exp Med Biol.* 2008;609:108-130
Exclusion code: 7

Machado ACS, Guimaraes EMB, Sakurai E, Fioravante FCR, Amaral WN, Alves MFC. High titers of Chlamydia trachomatis antibodies in Brazilian women with tubal occlusion or previous ectopic pregnancy. *Infect Dis Obstet Gynecol.* 2007;2007:24816
Exclusion code: 5

Madeleine MM, Anttila T, Schwartz SM, et al. Risk of cervical cancer associated with Chlamydia trachomatis antibodies by histology, HPV type and HPV cofactors. *Int J Cancer.* 2007;120(3):650-655
Exclusion code: 5

Magnus M, Schillinger JA, Fortenberry JD, Berman SM, Kissinger P. Partner age not associated with recurrent Chlamydia trachomatis infection, condom use, or partner treatment and referral among adolescent women. *J Adolesc Health.* 2006;39(3):396-403
Exclusion code: 5

Mahilum-Tapay L, Laitila V, Wawrzyniak JJ, et al. New point of care Chlamydia Rapid Test--bridging the gap between diagnosis and treatment: performance evaluation study. *BMJ.* 2007;335(7631):1190-1194
Exclusion code: 4

Mahmud NU, Hossain MA, Nahar K, et al. Non-culture diagnosis of Chlamydia trachomatis genital infection in sexually active women. *Mymensingh Med J.* 2012;21(1):8-12
Exclusion code: 11

Mahony JB, Jang D, Chong S, et al. Detection of Chlamydia trachomatis, Neisseria gonorrhoeae, Ureaplasma urealyticum, and Mycoplasma genitalium in First-void Urine Specimens by Multiplex Polymerase Chain Reaction. *Mol Diagn.* 1997;2(3):161-168
Exclusion code: 3

Mahto M, Mallinson H. Should we consider alternatives to combined cervical and urethral swabs for detection of Chlamydia trachomatis in females? *Sex Transm Infect.* 2007;83(4):335-336
Exclusion code: 3

Malenie R, Joshi PJ, Mathur MD. Chlamydia trachomatis antigen detection in pregnancy and its verification by antibody blocking assay. *Indian J.* 2006;24(2):97-100
Exclusion code: 5

Malik A, Jain S, Rizvi M, Shukla I, Hakim S. Chlamydia trachomatis infection in women with secondary infertility. *Fertil Steril.* 2009;91(1):91-95
Exclusion code: 3

Mangin D, Murdoch D, Wells JE, et al. Chlamydia trachomatis testing sensitivity in midstream compared with first-void urine specimens. *Ann Fam Med.* 2012;10(1):50-53
Exclusion code: 5

Manhart LE, Aral SO, Holmes KK, et al. Influence of study population on the identification of risk factors for sexually transmitted diseases using a case-control design: the example of gonorrhea. *Am J Epidemiol.* 2004;160(4):393-402
Exclusion code: 5

Manhas A, Sethi S, Sharma M, et al. Association of genital mycoplasmas including Mycoplasma genitalium in HIV infected men with nongonococcal urethritis attending STD & HIV clinics. *Indian J Med Res.* 2009;129(3):305-310

Appendix B4. Excluded Studies

Exclusion code: 3

Mann JR, McDermott S, Gill T. Sexually transmitted infection is associated with increased risk of preterm birth in South Carolina women insured by Medicaid. *J Matern Fetal Neonatal Med.* 2010;23(6):563-568
Exclusion code: 5

Marangoni A, Foschi C, Nardini P, et al. Evaluation of the new test VERSANT CT/GC DNA 1.0 assay for the detection of Chlamydia trachomatis and Neisseria gonorrhoeae in urine specimens. *J Clin Lab Anal.* 2012;26(2):70-72
Exclusion code: 4

Marcus JL, Bernstein KT, Kohn RP, Liska S, Philip SS. Infections missed by urethral-only screening for chlamydia or gonorrhea detection among men who have sex with men. *Sex Transm Dis.* 2011;38(10):922-924
Exclusion code: 2

Marin Gabriel MA, de las Heras Ibarra S, Bergon Sendin E, et al. [Respiratory infection due to Chlamydia trachomatis in infants. Clinical presentation and outcome in 18 patients]. *An Pediatr (Barc).* 2004;60(4):349-353
Exclusion code: 5

Markos AR. Testing asymptomatic heterosexual men for gonorrhoea. *Int J STD AIDS.* 2010;21(4):302
Exclusion code: 7

Marrazzo JM, Johnson RE, Green TA, et al. Impact of patient characteristics on performance of nucleic acid amplification tests and DNA probe for detection of Chlamydia trachomatis in women with genital infections. *J Clin Microbiol.* 2005;43(2):577-584
Exclusion code: 3

Marrazzo JM, Scholes D. Acceptability of urine-based screening for Chlamydia trachomatis in asymptomatic young men: a systematic review. *Sex Transm Dis.* 2008;35(11 Suppl):S28-33
Exclusion code: 5

Marshall R, Chernesky M, Jang D, et al. Characteristics of the m2000 automated sample preparation and multiplex real-time PCR system for detection of Chlamydia trachomatis and Neisseria gonorrhoeae. *J Clin Microbiol.* 2007;45(3):747-751
Exclusion code: 4

Martens MG, Fine P, Fuller D, et al. Clinical evaluation of a new Pap test-based method for screening of Chlamydia trachomatis and Neisseria gonorrhoeae using liquid-based cytology media. *South Med J.* 2013;106(9):506-512
Exclusion code: 3

Martin DH, Nsuami M, Schachter J, et al. Use of multiple nucleic acid amplification tests to define the infected-patient "gold standard" in clinical trials of new diagnostic tests for Chlamydia trachomatis infections. *J Clin Microbiol.* 2004;42(10):4749-4758
Exclusion code: 5

Masek BJ, Arora N, Quinn N, et al. Performance of three nucleic acid amplification tests for detection of Chlamydia trachomatis and Neisseria gonorrhoeae by use of self-collected vaginal swabs obtained via an Internet-based screening program. *J Clin Microbiol.* 2009;47(6):1663-1667
Exclusion code: 4

Mayor S. Chlamydia screening in young people fails to reduce prevalence. *BMJ.* 2009;339:b4736
Exclusion code: 7

McClure JB, Scholes D, Grothaus L, et al. Chlamydia screening in at-risk adolescent females: an evaluation of screening practices and modifiable screening correlates. *J Adolesc Health.* 2006;38(6):726-733
Exclusion code: 3

McDonnell DD, Levy V, Morton TJM. Risk factors for Chlamydia among young women in a northern california juvenile detention facility: implications for community intervention. *Sex Transm Dis.* 2009;36(2 Suppl):S29-33
Exclusion code: 5

McGowin CL, Whitlock GC, Pyles RB. High-throughput multistrain polymerase chain reaction quantification of Chlamydia trachomatis from clinical and preclinical urogenital specimens. *Diagn Microbiol Infect Dis.* 2009;64(2):117-123
Exclusion code: 4

McGrath CM, Katz AR, Lee MVC, Rochat RW. Chlamydia screening of adolescent females: a survey of providers in Hawaii. *J Community Health.* 2011;36(2):274-280
Exclusion code: 3

McMillan A, Manavi K, Young H. Concurrent gonococcal and chlamydial infections among men attending a sexually transmitted diseases clinic. *Int J STD AIDS.* 2005;16(5):357-361
Exclusion code: 5

Appendix B4. Excluded Studies

McMillan HM, O'Carroll H, Lambert JS, et al. Screening for Chlamydia trachomatis in asymptomatic women attending outpatient clinics in a large maternity hospital in Dublin, Ireland. *Sex Transm Infect.* 2006;82(6):503-505
Exclusion code: 5

McNally LP, Templeton DJ, Jin F, et al. Low positive predictive value of a nucleic acid amplification test for nongenital Neisseria gonorrhoeae infection in homosexual men. *Clin Infect Dis.* 2008;47(2):e25-27
Exclusion code: 4

McNulty CAM, Freeman E, Howell-Jones R, et al. Overcoming the barriers to chlamydia screening in general practice--a qualitative study. *Fam Pract.* 2010;27(3):291-302
Exclusion code: 3

McNulty CAM, Hogan AH, Ricketts EJ, et al. Increasing chlamydia screening tests in general practice: a modified Zelen prospective Cluster Randomised Controlled Trial evaluating a complex intervention based on the Theory of Planned Behaviour. *Sex Transm Infect.* 2014;90(3):188-194
Exclusion code: 4

Meader E, Waters J, Sillis M. Chlamydia trachomatis RNA in the environment: is there potential for false-positive nucleic acid amplification test results? *Sex Transm Infect.* 2008;84(2):107-110
Exclusion code: 5

Merz AJ, So M. Interactions of pathogenic Neisseriae with epithelial cell membranes. *Annu Rev Cell Dev Biol.* 2000;16:423-457
Exclusion code: 2

Mevissen FEF, Meertens RM, Ruiter RAC, Feenstra H, Schaalma HP. HIV/STI risk communication: the effects of scenario-based risk information and frequency-based risk information on perceived susceptibility to chlamydia and HIV. *J Health Psychol.* 2009;14(1):78-87
Exclusion code: 4

Meyers D, Wolff T, Gregory K, et al. USPSTF recommendations for STI screening. *Am Fam Physician.* 2008;77(6):819-824
Exclusion code: 2

Meyers DS, Halvorson H, Luckhaupt S. Screening for Chlamydial Infection: A Focused Evidence Update for the U.S. Preventive Services Task Force. Rockville (MD): *Agency for Healthcare Research and Quality*; Jun Preventive Services Task Force 2007Exclusion code: 2

Meyers DS, Halvorson H, Luckhaupt S, Force USPST. Screening for chlamydial infection: an evidence update for the U.S. Preventive Services Task Force. *Ann Intern Med.* 2007;147(2):135-142
Exclusion code: 2

Michaud DS, Platz EA, Giovannucci E. Gonorrhoea and male bladder cancer in a prospective study. *Br J Cancer.* 2007;96(1):169-171
Exclusion code: 5

Michel C-EC, Sonnex C, Carne CA, et al. Chlamydia trachomatis load at matched anatomic sites: implications for screening strategies. *J Clin Microbiol.* 2007;45(5):1395-1402
Exclusion code: 5

Miller JM, Maupin RT, Nsuami M. Initial and repeat testing for chlamydia during pregnancy. *J Matern Fetal Neonatal Med.* 2005;18(4):231-235
Exclusion code: 5

Miller KE. Diagnosis and treatment of Neisseria gonorrhoeae infections. *Am Fam Physician.* 2006;73(10):1779-1784
Exclusion code: 7

Miller KE. Diagnosis and treatment of Chlamydia trachomatis infection. *Am Fam Physician.* 2006;73(8):1411-1416
Exclusion code: 7

Miller WC. Screening for chlamydial infection: are we doing enough? *Lancet.* 2005;365(9458):456-458
Exclusion code: 7

Miller WC, Hoffman IF, Owen-O'Dowd J, et al. Selective screening for chlamydial infection: which criteria to use? *Am J Prev Med.* 2000;18(2):115-122
Exclusion code: 2

Mills N, Daker-White G, Graham A, Campbell R. Population screening for Chlamydia trachomatis infection in the UK: a qualitative study of the experiences of those screened. *Fam Pract.* 2006;23(5):550-557
Exclusion code: 6

Miranda AE, Szwarcwald CL, Peres RL, Page-Shafer K. Prevalence and risk behaviors for chlamydial infection in a population-based study of female adolescents in Brazil. *Sex Transm Dis.* 2004;31(9):542-546

Appendix B4. Excluded Studies

Exclusion code: 5

Mitka M. CDC: improve targeted screening for chlamydia. *Jama.* 2012;307(14):1472
Exclusion code: 7

Molano M, Meijer CJLM, Morre SA, Pol R, van den Brule AJC. Combination of PCR targeting the VD2 of omp1 and reverse line blot analysis for typing of urogenital Chlamydia trachomatis serovars in cervical scrape specimens. *J Clin Microbiol.* 2004;42(7):2935-2939
Exclusion code: 4

Moller JK, Pedersen LN, Persson K. Comparison of Gen-probe transcription-mediated amplification, Abbott PCR, and Roche PCR assays for detection of wild-type and mutant plasmid strains of Chlamydia trachomatis in Sweden. *J Clin Microbiol.* 2008;46(12):3892-3895
Exclusion code: 5

Moller JK, Pedersen LN, Persson K. Comparison of the Abbott RealTime CT new formulation assay with two other commercial assays for detection of wild-type and new variant strains of Chlamydia trachomatis. *J Clin Microbiol.* 2010;48(2):440-443
Exclusion code: 3

Moncada J, Donegan E, Schachter J. Evaluation of CDC-recommended approaches for confirmatory testing of positive Neisseria gonorrhoeae nucleic acid amplification test results. *J Clin Microbiol.* 2008;46(5):1614-1619
Exclusion code: 4

Moncada J, Schachter J, Liska S, Shayevich C, Klausner JD. Evaluation of self-collected glans and rectal swabs from men who have sex with men for detection of Chlamydia trachomatis and Neisseria gonorrhoeae by use of nucleic acid amplification tests. *J Clin Microbiol.* 2009;47(6):1657-1662
Exclusion code: 4

Morgan J, Donnell A, Bell A. Does a clinical guideline change chlamydia testing? Report from the Waikato Chlamydia Project. *J Prim Health Care.* 2012;4(1):45-51
Exclusion code: 5

Morris SR, Bauer HM, Chartier M, et al. Relative efficiency of chlamydia screening in non-clinical settings in two California counties. *Int J STD AIDS.* 2010;21(1):52-56
Exclusion code: 5

Morris W, Omokanye S. Chlamydia rates in postcoital IUD recipients. *J Fam Plann Reprod Health Care.* 2006;32(3):204
Exclusion code: 7

Morton AN, Wakefield T, Tabrizi SN, Garland SM, Fairley CK. An outreach programme for sexually transmitted infection screening in street sex workers using self-administered samples. *Int J STD AIDS.* 1999;10(11):741-743
Exclusion code: 5

Moss S, Mallinson H. The contribution of APTIMA Combo 2 assay to the diagnosis of gonorrhoea in genitourinary medicine setting. *Int J STD AIDS.* 2007;18(8):551-554
Exclusion code: 3

Moss TR, Van Der Pol B. Dual infection with Neisseria gonorrhoeae and Chlamydia trachomatis. *Int J STD AIDS.* 2009;20(2):143-144
Exclusion code: 7

Mossenson A, Algie K, Olding M, Garton L, Reeve C. 'Yes wee can' - a nurse-driven asymptomatic screening program for chlamydia and gonorrhoea in a remote emergency department. *Sex Health.* 2012;9(2):194-195
Exclusion code: 10

Mukherjee A, Sood S, Bala M, et al. The role of a commercial enzyme immuno assay antigen detection system for diagnosis of C. trachomatis in genital swab samples. *Indian J.* 2011;29(4):411-413
Exclusion code: 3

Mundy L, Hiller J. Rapid point-of-care test for the detection of Chlamydia in individuals at risk of trachoma. National Horizon Scanning Unit 2006;13(1).
Exclusion code: 7

Opportunistic screening of symptomatic individuals for Chlamydia Commonwealth of Australia 2007.
Exclusion code: 7

Munson E, Boyd V, Czarnecka J, et al. Evaluation of Gen-Probe APTIMA-based Neisseria gonorrhoeae and Chlamydia trachomatis confirmatory testing in a metropolitan setting of high disease prevalence. *J Clin Microbiol.* 2007;45(9):2793-2797
Exclusion code: 4

Murphy PA, Jacobson J, Turok DK. Criterion-based screening for sexually transmitted infection: sensitivity, specificity, and predictive values of

commonly used questions. *J Midwifery Womens Health.* 2012;57(6):622-628
Exclusion code: 4

Mushanski LM, Brandt K, Coffin N, Levett PN, Horsman GB, Rank EL. Comparison of the BD Viper System with XTR Technology to the Gen-Probe APTIMA COMBO 2 Assay using the TIGRIS DTS system for the detection of Chlamydia trachomatis and Neisseria gonorrhoeae in urine specimens. *Sex Transm Dis.* 2012;39(7):514-517
Exclusion code: 3

Myziuk L, Romanowski B, Brown M. Endocervical Gram stain smears and their usefulness in the diagnosis of Chlamydia trachomatis. *Sex Transm Infect.* 2001;77(2):103-106
Exclusion code: 3

Nadala E-C, Goh BT, Magbanua J-P, et al. Performance evaluation of a new rapid urine test for chlamydia in men: prospective cohort study. *BMJ.* 2009;339:b2655
Exclusion code: 4

Nagasawa Z, Ikeda-Dantsuji Y, Niwa T, Miyakoshi H, Nagayama A. Evaluation of APTIMA Combo 2 for cross-reactivity with oropharyngeal Neisseria species and other microorganisms. *Clin Chim Acta.* 2010;411(9-10):776-778
Exclusion code: 5

Nasution TA, Cheong SF, Lim CT, Leong EWK, Ngeow YF. Multiplex PCR for the detection of urogenital pathogens in mothers and newborns. *Malays J Pathol.* 2007;29(1):19-24
Exclusion code: 3

Naucler P, Chen H-C, Persson K, et al. Seroprevalence of human papillomaviruses and Chlamydia trachomatis and cervical cancer risk: nested case-control study. *J Gen Virol.* 2007;88(Pt 3):814-822
Exclusion code: 5

Nelson H, Cantor A, Zakher B, Fraenkel M, Pappas M. Screening for Gonorhea and Chlamydia: Systematic Review to Update the U.S. Preventive Services Task Force Recommendations [in press]. Rockvile, MD: Agency for Healthcare Research and Quality2014Exclusion code: 2

Nelson HD, Helfand M. Screening for chlamydial infection. *Am J Prev Med.* 2001;20(3 SUPPL.):95-107
Exclusion code: 2

Ness RB, Shen C, Bass D, et al. Chlamydia trachomatis serology in women with and without ovarian cancer. *Infect Dis Obstet Gynecol.* 2008;2008:219672
Exclusion code: 5

Ness RB, Smith KJ, Chang C-CH, Schisterman EF, Bass DC, Gynecologic Infection Follow-Through GI. Prediction of pelvic inflammatory disease among young, single, sexually active women. *Sex Transm Dis.* 2006;33(3):137-142
Exclusion code: 5

Nogales MC, Castro C, Ramirez M, et al. [Diagnosis of Chlamydia trachomatis infection in a clinic for sexually transmitted disease: evaluation of cervical, urethral and rectal swab samples by polymerase chain reaction]. *Enferm Infecc Microbiol Clin.* 2007;25(1):11-15
Exclusion code: 3

Noguchi Y, Kanyama A, Fujita M, et al. [Evaluation of the new nucleic acid amplification system for direct detection of Chlamydia trachomatis and Neisseria gonorrhoeae in women]. *Kansenshogaku Zasshi.* 2006;80(3):251-256
Exclusion code: 8

Noone A, Spiers A, Allardice G, et al. Opportunistic screening for genital Chlamydia trachomatis infection and partner follow-up in family planning clinics in three Scottish cities. *J Fam Plann Reprod Health Care.* 2004;30(2):84-85
Exclusion code: 10

Novak D, Novak M. Use of the Internet for home testing for Chlamydia trachomatis in Sweden: who are the users? *Int J STD AIDS.* 2012;23(2):83-87
Exclusion code: 4

Novak DP, Karlsson RB. Simplifying chlamydia testing: an innovative Chlamydia trachomatis testing approach using the internet and a home sampling strategy: population based study. *Sex Transm Infect.* 2006;82(2):142-147; discussion 152-143
Exclusion code: 10

Oakeshott P, Aghaizu A, Reid F, et al. Frequency and risk factors for prevalent, incident, and persistent genital carcinogenic human papillomavirus infection in sexually active women: community based cohort study. *BMJ.* 2012;344:e4168
Exclusion code: 5

Oakeshott P, Kerry S, Atherton H, et al. Community-based trial of screening for Chlamydia trachomatis to

prevent pelvic inflammatory disease: The POPI (Prevention Of Pelvic Infection) Trial. *Trials.* 2008;9
Exclusion code: 7

Okuda H, Ohya K, Shiota Y, Kato H, Fukushi H. Detection of Chlamydophila psittaci by using SYBR green real-time PCR. *J Vet Med Sci.* 2011;73(2):249-254
Exclusion code: 3

Oliveira MdL, Amorim MMRd, Souza ASRd, Albuquerque LCBd, Costa AARd. [Chlamydia infection in patients with and without cervical intra-epithelial lesions]. *Rev Assoc Med Bras.* 2008;54(6):506-512
Exclusion code: 5

Oliveira MdL, Amorim MMRd, Souza PREd, Albuquerque LCBd, Brandao LAC, Guimaraes RL. Chlamydia infection in patients with and without cervical intra-epithelial lesions tested by real-time PCR vs. direct immunofluorescence. *Braz J Infect Dis.* 2008;12(4):324-328
Exclusion code: 5

Olshen E, Shrier LA. Diagnostic tests for chlamydial and gonorrheal infections. *Semin Pediatr Infect Dis.* 2005;16(3):192-198
Exclusion code: 7

O'Mahony C, Gupta M, Edirisinghe D, Worthen E. One-year experience of APTIMA COMBO 2 Transcription Mediated Assay (TMA) for chlamydia and gonorrhoea in a district general hospital. *Int J STD AIDS.* 2006;17(4):283
Exclusion code: 6

O'Mahony C, Reeve-Fowkes A, Worthen E, Mallinson H. Three years of using Aptima Combo 2 (AC2) transcription-mediated amplification for gonorrhoea in a district hospital genitourinary medicine clinic shows it to be superior to culture and has a specificity of almost 100%. *Int J STD AIDS.* 2008;19(1):67-69
Exclusion code: 7

O'Neil D, Doseeva V, Rothmann T, Wolff J, Nazarenko I. Evaluation of Chlamydia trachomatis and Neisseria gonorrhoeae detection in urine, endocervical, and vaginal specimens by a multiplexed isothermal thermophilic helicase-dependent amplification (tHDA) assay. *J Clin Microbiol.* 2011;49(12):4121-4125
Exclusion code: 4

Oppelt P, Renner SP, Strick R, et al. Correlation of high-risk human papilloma viruses but not of herpes viruses or Chlamydia trachomatis with endometriosis lesions. *Fertil Steril.* 2010;93(6):1778-1786
Exclusion code: 5

Ostergaard L, Andersen B, Moller JK, Olesen F. Home sampling versus conventional swab sampling for screening of Chlamydia trachomatis in women: a cluster-randomized 1-year follow-up study. *Clin Infect Dis.* 2000;31(4):951-957
Exclusion code: 3

Ostergaard L, Andersen B, Olesen F, Moller JK. Efficacy of home sampling for screening of Chlamydia trachomatis: randomised study. *BMJ.* 1998;317(7150):26-27
Exclusion code: 3

Ostergaard L, Moller JK, Andersen B, Olesen F. Diagnosis of urogenital Chlamydia trachomatis infection in women based on mailed samples obtained at home: multipractice comparative study. *BMJ.* 1996;313(7066):1186-1189
Exclusion code: 3

Ota KV, Tamari IE, Smieja M, et al. Detection of Neisseria gonorrhoeae and Chlamydia trachomatis in pharyngeal and rectal specimens using the BD Probetec ET system, the Gen-Probe Aptima Combo 2 assay and culture. *Sex Transm Infect.* 2009;85(3):182-186
Exclusion code: 3

Ouden DD, Derouin A, Silva S, Khan A. Screening for chlamydia: are you doing it? *Nurse Pract.* 2014;39(4):41-47
Exclusion code: 7

Owusu-Edusei K, Bohm MK, Kent CK. Diagnostic methodologies for chlamydia screening in females aged 15 to 25 years from private insurance claims data in the United States, 2001 to 2005. *Sex Transm Dis.* 2009;36(7):419-421
Exclusion code: 10

Paavonen J. [Chlamydia carrier--symptomless or unfaithful?]. *Duodecim.* 2012;128(13):1351-1356
Exclusion code: 8

Palmer HM, Gilroy CB, Thomas BJ, Hay PE, Gilchrist C, Taylor-Robinson D. Detection of Chlamydia trachomatis by the polymerase chain reaction in swabs and urine from men with non-gonococcal urethritis. *J Clin Pathol.* 1991;44(4):321-325

Appendix B4. Excluded Studies

Exclusion code: 3

Panknin H-T. [How frequently are chlamydia responsible for newborn conjunctivitis? A study in Holland reveals current prevalence]. *Kinderkrankenschwester.* 2009;28(7):294-295
Exclusion code: 8

Papp JR, Ahrens K, Phillips C, Kent CK, Philip S, Klausner JD. The use and performance of oral-throat rinses to detect pharyngeal Neisseria gonorrhoeae and Chlamydia trachomatis infections. *Diagn Microbiol Infect Dis.* 2007;59(3):259-264
Exclusion code: 4

Park J, Marcus JL, Pandori M, Snell A, Philip SS, Bernstein KT. Sentinel surveillance for pharyngeal chlamydia and gonorrhea among men who have sex with men--San Francisco, 2010. *Sex Transm Dis.* 2012;39(6):482-484
Exclusion code: 5

Parra-Sanchez M, Palomares JC, Bernal S, et al. Evaluation of the cobas 4800 CT/NG Test for detecting Chlamydia trachomatis and Neisseria gonorrhoeae DNA in urogenital swabs and urine specimens. *Diagn Microbiol Infect Dis.* 2012;74(4):338-342
Exclusion code: 3

Pathela P, Hennessy RR, Blank S, Parvez F, Franklin W, Schillinger JA. The contribution of a urine-based jail screening program to citywide male Chlamydia and gonorrhea case rates in New York City. *Sex Transm Dis.* 2009;36(2 Suppl):S58-61
Exclusion code: 5

Pearce DM, Shenton DP, Holden J, Gaydos CA. Evaluation of a novel electrochemical detection method for Chlamydia trachomatis: application for point-of-care diagnostics. *IEEE Trans Biomed Eng.* 2011;58(3):755-758
Exclusion code: 4

Peng X-b, Zeng K. Ligase chain reaction for Chlamydia trachomatis detection in urine specimens from symptomatic and asymptomatic men. *Di Yi Jun Yi Da Xue Xue Bao.* 2004;24(5):485-488
Exclusion code: 4

Penney GC, Thomson M, Norman J, et al. A randomised comparison of strategies for reducing infective complications of induced abortion. *Br J Obstet Gynaecol.* 1998;105(6):599-604
Exclusion code: 4

Perlik M, Drews K, Pienskowski W. Is it justifiable to perform screening tests for Chlamydia trachomatis in pregnant women? *Med Wieku Rozwoj.* 2005;9(1):117-125
Exclusion code: 7

Perquin DAM, Beersma MFC, de Craen AJM, Helmerhorst FM. The value of Chlamydia trachomatis-specific IgG antibody testing and hysterosalpingography for predicting tubal pathology and occurrence of pregnancy. *Fertil Steril.* 2007;88(1):224-226
Exclusion code: 5

Peterman TA, Newman DR, Goldberg M, et al. Screening male prisoners for Chlamydia trachomatis: impact on test positivity among women from their neighborhoods who were tested in family planning clinics. *Sex Transm Dis.* 2009;36(7):425-429
Exclusion code: 5

Petersen RW, Tabrizi SN, Garland S, Quinlivan JA. Prevalence of Chlamydia trachomatis in a public colposcopy clinic population. *Sex Health.* 2007;4(2):133-136
Exclusion code: 5

Pientong C, Ekalaksananan T, Wonglikitpanya N, Swadpanich U, Kongyingyoes B, Kleebkaow P. Chlamydia trachomatis infections and the risk of ectopic pregnancy in Khon Kaen women. *J Obstet Gynaecol Res.* 2009;35(4):775-781
Exclusion code: 5

Pittaras TE, Papaparaskevas J, Houhoula DP, et al. Comparison of penile skin swab with intra-urethral swab and first void urine for polymerase chain reaction-based diagnosis of Chlamydia trachomatis urethritis in male patients. *Sex Transm Dis.* 2008;35(12):999-1001
Exclusion code: 4

Pope CF, Hay P, Alexander S, et al. Positive predictive value of the Becton Dickinson VIPER system and the ProbeTec GC Q x assay, in extracted mode, for detection of Neisseria gonorrhoeae. *Sex Transm Infect.* 2010;86(6):465-469
Exclusion code: 3

Porter KA, Thomas JC, Emch ME. Variations in the effect of incarceration on community gonorrhea rates, Guilford County, North Carolina, 2005-2006. *Int J STD AIDS.* 2010;21(1):34-38
Exclusion code: 5

Appendix B4. Excluded Studies

Potterat JJ. Active detection of men with asymptomatic chlamydial or gonorrhoeal urethritis. *Int J STD AIDS.* 2005;16(6):458
Exclusion code: 7

Powers ME, Adekeye T, Volny R. Chlamydia screening: what about the men? *Am J Public Health.* 2011;101(4):583-584; author reply 584-585
Exclusion code: 7

Public Health Agency of Canada. Canadian Guidelines on Sexually Transmitted Infections,2010Exclusion code: 2
Public Health Agency of Canada. Canadian Guidelines on Sexually Transmitted Infections. Section 5 - Management and Treatment of Specific Infections; Gonococcal Infections: Revised July 2013 2013; http://www.phac-aspc.gc.ca/std-mts/sti-its/cgsti-ldcits/section-5-6-eng.php#toc361210448Exclusion code: 2.

Quint KD, Bom RJM, Bruisten SM, et al. Comparison of three genotyping methods to identify Chlamydia trachomatis genotypes in positive men and women. *Mol Cell Probes.* 2010;24(5):266-270
Exclusion code: 4

Radouani F, Maile J, Betsou F. Serological profiling with Chlamycheck, a commercial multiplex recombinant antigen Western blot assay of chlamydial infections. *Can J Microbiol.* 2007;53(12):1360-1368
Exclusion code: 3

Rahman MS, Beever W, Skov S, Boffa J. Using urinary leucocyte esterase tests as an indicator of infection with gonorrhoea or chlamydia in asymptomatic males in a primary health care setting. *Int J STD AIDS.* 2014;25(2):138-144
Exclusion code: 4

Rank EL, Sautter RL, Beavis KG, et al. A two-site analytical evaluation of the BD Viper System with XTR Technology in Nonextracted Mode and Extracted Mode with seeded simulated specimens. *J Lab Autom.* 2011;16(4):271-275
Exclusion code: 4

Raychaudhuri M, Birley HDL. Audit of routine rectal swabs for gonorrhoea culture in women. *Int J STD AIDS.* 2010;21(2):143-144
Exclusion code: 5

Razali MF, Fairley CK, Hocking J, Bradshaw CS, Chen MY. Sampling technique and detection rates for pharyngeal gonorrhea using culture. *Sex Transm Dis.* 2010;37(8):522-524
Exclusion code: 5

Reagan MM, Xu H, Shih SL, Secura GM, Peipert JF. A randomized trial of home versus clinic-based sexually transmitted disease screening among men. *Sex Transm Dis.* 2012;39(11):842-847
Exclusion code: 5

Regua-Mangia AH, Brito CMMd, Rosa RS, Correa MA, Santos-Perisse AR. Molecular diagnosis and genotyping of Neisseria gonorrhoeae in urine samples from women at low-income communities in Rio de Janeiro, Brazil. *Braz J Infect Dis.* 2012;16(1):105-106
Exclusion code: 3

Reid RJ, Scholes D, Grothaus L, et al. Is provider continuity associated with chlamydia screening for adolescent and young adult women? *Prev Med.* 2005;41(5-6):865-872
Exclusion code: 5

Renton A, Filatova E, Ison C, et al. Performance of direct fluorescent antibody tests for routine diagnosis of Chlamydia trachomatis in Russian sexually transmitted disease clinics. *Int J STD AIDS.* 2008;19(12):851-855
Exclusion code: 4

Renton A, Filatova E, Ison C, et al. A trial of the validity of genital smears and cultures with gonococcal vaccine provocation in diagnosing genital gonorrhoea in women. *Int J STD AIDS.* 2009;20(1):24-29
Exclusion code: 4

Renton A, Thomas BM, Gill S, Lowndes C, Taylor-Robinson D, Patterson K. Chlamydia trachomatis in cervical and vaginal swabs and urine specimens from women undergoing termination of pregnancy. *Int J STD AIDS.* 2006;17(7):443-447
Exclusion code: 3

Richardus JH, Gotz HM. Risk selection and targeted interventions in community-based control of chlamydia. *Curr Opin Infect Dis.* 2007;20(1):60-65
Exclusion code: 6

Rietmeijer CA, Hopkins E, Geisler WM, Orr DP, Kent CK. Chlamydia trachomatis positivity rates among men tested in selected venues in the United States: a review of the recent literature. *Sex Transm Dis.* 2008;35(11 Suppl):S8-S18
Exclusion code: 5

Appendix B4. Excluded Studies

Roberts CH, Last A, Molina-Gonzalez S, et al. Development and evaluation of a next-generation digital PCR diagnostic assay for ocular Chlamydia trachomatis infections. *J Clin Microbiol.* 2013;51(7):2195-2203
Exclusion code: 4

Roberts SW, Sheffield JS, McIntire DD, Alexander JM. Urine screening for Chlamydia trachomatis during pregnancy. *Obstet Gynecol.* 2011;117(4):883-885
Exclusion code: 3

Rockett R, Goire N, Limnios A, et al. Evaluation of the cobas 4800 CT/NG test for detecting Chlamydia trachomatis and Neisseria gonorrhoeae. *Sex Transm Infect.* 2010;86(6):470-473
Exclusion code: 3

Rompalo AM, Gaydos CA, Shah N, et al. Evaluation of use of a single intravaginal swab to detect multiple sexually transmitted infections in active-duty military women. *Clin Infect Dis.* 2001;33(9):1455-1461
Exclusion code: 3

Rose SB, Lawton BA, Bromhead C, MacDonald EJ, Elley CR. Poor uptake of self-sample collection kits for Chlamydia testing outside primary care. *Aust N Z J Public Health.* 2010;34(5):517-520
Exclusion code: 5

Rosenthal DA, Fairley CK, Garland SM, et al. Homeless young people: an important risk group for sexually transmitted infections. *Med J Aust.* 2000;172(5):244
Exclusion code: 5

Ross JDC, Radcliffe KW. Why do those using illicit drugs have higher rates of sexually transmitted infection? *Int J STD AIDS.* 2006;17(4):247-253
Exclusion code: 5

Roth A, Van Der Pol B, Dodge B, Fortenberry JD, Zimet G. Future chlamydia screening preferences of men attending a sexually transmissible infection clinic. *Sex Health.* 2011;8(3):419-426
Exclusion code: 4

Røttingen JA, Cameron WD, Garnett GP. A systematic review of the epidemiologic interactions between classic sexually transmitted diseases and HIV: How much really is known? *Sex Transm Dis.* 2001;28(10):579-597
Exclusion code: 2

Rours GIJG, Duijts L, Moll HA, et al. Chlamydia trachomatis infection during pregnancy associated with preterm delivery: a population-based prospective cohort study. *Eur J Epidemiol.* 2011;26(6):493-502
Exclusion code: 10

Rours GIJG, Verkooyen RP, Willemse HFM, et al. Use of pooled urine samples and automated DNA isolation to achieve improved sensitivity and cost-effectiveness of large-scale testing for Chlamydia trachomatis in pregnant women. *J Clin Microbiol.* 2005;43(9):4684-4690
Exclusion code: 4

Rowhani-Rahbar A, Niccolai LM, Dunne DW, Green S, Jenkins H, Khoshnood K. Comparative epidemiology of Chlamydia trachomatis infection among men attending sexually transmitted disease clinics with and without indication for testing. *Int J STD AIDS.* 2006;17(7):453-458
Exclusion code: 5

Ruhl C. Update on Chlamydia and gonorrhea screening during pregnancy. *Nurs Womens Health.* 2013;17(2):143-146
Exclusion code: 7

Ryan C, Kudesia G, McIntyre S, Davies S, Zadik P, Kinghorn GR. BD ProbeTec ET assay for the diagnosis of gonorrhoea in a high-risk population: a protocol for replacing traditional microscopy and culture techniques. *Sex Transm Infect.* 2007;83(3):175-179; discussion 179-180
Exclusion code: 3

Ryder N, Lockart IG, Bourne C. Is screening asymptomatic men who have sex with men for urethral gonorrhoea worthwhile? *Sex Health.* 2010;7(1):90-91
Exclusion code: 5

Sabido M, Hernandez G, Gonzalez V, et al. Clinic-based evaluation of a rapid point-of-care test for detection of Chlamydia trachomatis in specimens from sex workers in Escuintla, Guatemala. *J Clin Microbiol.* 2009;47(2):475-476
Exclusion code: 4

Sachse K, Hotzel H, Slickers P, Ehricht R. The use of DNA microarray technology for detection and genetic characterisation of chlamydiae. *Dev Biol (Basel).* 2006;126:203-210; discussion 326-207
Exclusion code: 5

Appendix B4. Excluded Studies

Sachse K, Hotzel H, Slickers P, Ellinger T, Ehricht R. DNA microarray-based detection and identification of Chlamydia and Chlamydophila spp. *Mol Cell Probes.* 2005;19(1):41-50
Exclusion code: 3

Safaeian M, Quint K, Schiffman M, et al. Chlamydia trachomatis and risk of prevalent and incident cervical premalignancy in a population-based cohort. *J Natl Cancer Inst.* 2010;102(23):1794-1804
Exclusion code: 5

Salazar LF, Crosby RA, Diclemente RJ. Exploring the mediating mechanism between gender-based violence and biologically confirmed Chlamydia among detained adolescent girls. *Violence Against Women.* 2009;15(3):258-275
Exclusion code: 5

Salerno J, Darling-Fisher C, Hawkins NM, Fraker E. Identifying relationships between high-risk sexual behaviors and screening positive for chlamydia and gonorrhea in school-wide screening events. *J Sch Health.* 2013;83(2):99-104
Exclusion code: 5

Samarawickrama A, Alexander S, Ison C. A laboratory-based evaluation of the BioStar Optical ImmunoAssay point-of-care test for diagnosing Neisseria gonorrhoeae infection. *J Med Microbiol.* 2011;60(Pt 12):1779-1781
Exclusion code: 4

Samra Z, Rosenberg S, Madar-Shapiro L. Direct simultaneous detection of 6 sexually transmitted pathogens from clinical specimens by multiplex polymerase chain reaction and auto-capillary electrophoresis. *Diagn Microbiol Infect Dis.* 2011;70(1):17-21
Exclusion code: 3

Sarlangue J, Castella C. [Chlamydia infection in neonates and infants]. *Arch Pediatr.* 2005;12 Suppl 1:S32-34
Exclusion code: 8

Satterwhite CL, Gray AM, Berman S, Weinstock H, Kleinbaum D, Howards PP. Chlamydia trachomatis infections among women attending prenatal clinics: United States, 2004-2009. *Sex Transm Dis.* 2012;39(6):416-420
Exclusion code: 5

Satterwhite CL, Grier L, Patzer R, Weinstock H, Howards PP, Kleinbaum D. Chlamydia positivity trends among women attending family planning

clinics: United States, 2004-2008. *Sex Transm Dis.* 2011;38(11):989-994
Exclusion code: 8

Savage EJ, Hughes G, Ison C, Lowndes CM, European Surveillance of Sexually Transmitted Infections n. Syphilis and gonorrhoea in men who have sex with men: a European overview. *Euro Surveill.* 2009;14(47)
Exclusion code: 5

Schachter J, Chernesky MA, Willis DE, et al. Vaginal swabs are the specimens of choice when screening for Chlamydia trachomatis and Neisseria gonorrhoeae: results from a multicenter evaluation of the APTIMA assays for both infections. *Sex Transm Dis.* 2005;32(12):725-728
Exclusion code: 3

Schachter J, Chow JM, Howard H, Bolan G, Moncada J. Detection of Chlamydia trachomatis by nucleic acid amplification testing: our evaluation suggests that CDC-recommended approaches for confirmatory testing are ill-advised. *J Clin Microbiol.* 2006;44(7):2512-2517
Exclusion code: 4

Schachter J, Hook EW, Martin DH, et al. Confirming positive results of nucleic acid amplification tests (NAATs) for Chlamydia trachomatis: all NAATs are not created equal. *J Clin Microbiol.* 2005;43(3):1372-1373
Exclusion code: 4

Schachter J, Moncada J, Liska S, Shayevich C, Klausner JD. Nucleic acid amplification tests in the diagnosis of chlamydial and gonococcal infections of the oropharynx and rectum in men who have sex with men. *Sex Transm Dis.* 2008;35(7):637-642
Exclusion code: 2

Schembri G, Schober P. Risk factors for chlamydial infection in chlamydia contacts: a questionnaire-based study. *J Fam Plann Reprod Health Care.* 2011;37(1):10-16
Exclusion code: 3

Scholes D, Satterwhite CL, Yu O, Fine D, Weinstock H, Berman S. Long-term trends in Chlamydia trachomatis infections and related outcomes in a U.S. managed care population. *Sex Transm Dis.* 2012;39(2):81-88
Exclusion code: 10

Scholes D, Stergachis A, Heidrich FE, Andrilla H, Holmes KK, Stamm WE. Prevention of pelvic

Appendix B4. Excluded Studies

inflammatory disease by screening for cervical chlamydial infection. *N Engl J Med.* 1996;334(21):1362-1366
Exclusion code: 2

Schwartz RM, Hogben M, Liddon N, et al. Coping with a diagnosis of C trachomatis or N gonorrhoeae: psychosocial and behavioral correlates. *J Health Psychol.* 2008;13(7):921-929
Exclusion code: 3

Scott G. Chlamydia and male fertility. *J R Soc Promot Health.* 2004;124(5):211-212
Exclusion code: 7

Scragg S, Bingham A, Mallinson H. Should Chlamydia trachomatis confirmation make you cross? Performance of collection kits tested across three nucleic acid amplification test platforms. *Sex Transm Infect.* 2006;82(4):295-297
Exclusion code: 4

Sellors JW, Lorincz AT, Mahony JB, et al. Comparison of self-collected vaginal, vulvar and urine samples with physician-collected cervical samples for human papillomavirus testing to detect high-grade squamous intraepithelial lesions. *Cmaj.* 2000;163(5):513-518
Exclusion code: 5

Senior K. Chlamydia: a much underestimated STI. *Lancet Infect Dis.* 2012;12(7):517-518
Exclusion code: 7

Seth P, Wingood GM, DiClemente RJ, Robinson LS. Alcohol use as a marker for risky sexual behaviors and biologically confirmed sexually transmitted infections among young adult African-American women. *Womens Health Issues.* 2011;21(2):130-135
Exclusion code: 4

Sethupathi M, Blackwell A. Chlamydia trachomatis infection: the efficacy and safety of a fast-track referral and treatment system. *Int J STD AIDS.* 2009;20(3):184-187
Exclusion code: 5

Sexton ME, Baker JJ, Nakagawa K, et al. How reliable is self-testing for gonorrhea and chlamydia among men who have sex with men? *J Fam Pract.* 2013;62(2):70-78
Exclusion code: 5

Sharqi AA, Thompson C, Clutterbuck DJ. How many sexually transmitted infections (STIs) will we miss?--

an algorithm to assess risk factors for STI. *Int J STD AIDS.* 2006;17(8):558-559
Exclusion code: 3

She RC, Welch R, Wilson AR, Davis D, Litwin CM. Correlation of Chlamydia and Chlamydophila spp. IgG and IgM antibodies by microimmunofluorescence with antigen detection methods. *J Clin Lab Anal.* 2011;25(4):305-308
Exclusion code: 5

Sheffield JS, Andrews WW, Klebanoff MA, et al. Spontaneous resolution of asymptomatic Chlamydia trachomatis in pregnancy. *Obstet Gynecol.* 2005;105(3):557-562
Exclusion code: 5

Sheringham J. Screening for Chlamydia. *BMJ.* 2010;340:c1698
Exclusion code: 7

Sherley M, Kennedy KJ, Martin SJ. Screening with nucleic acid amplification tests for gonorrhoea in men who have sex with men. *Med J Aust.* 2012;197(6):332
Exclusion code: 7

Shields SA, Wong T, Mann J, et al. Prevalence and correlates of Chlamydia infection in Canadian street youth. *J Adolesc Health.* 2004;34(5):384-390
Exclusion code: 5

Shrier LA, Schillinger JA, Aneja P, et al. Depressive symptoms and sexual risk behavior in young, chlamydia-infected, heterosexual dyads. *J Adolesc Health.* 2009;45(1):63-69
Exclusion code: 3

Siemer J, Theile O, Larbi Y, et al. Chlamydia trachomatis infection as a risk factor for infertility among women in Ghana, West Africa. *Am J Trop Med Hyg.* 2008;78(2):323-327
Exclusion code: 5

Silva LCF, Miranda AE, Batalha RS, et al. Chlamydia trachomatis infection among HIV-infected women attending an AIDS clinic in the city of Manaus, Brazil. *Braz J Infect Dis.* 2012;16(4):335-338
Exclusion code: 3

Silva MJPMdA, Florencio GLD, Gabiatti JRE, Amaral RLd, Eleuterio Junior J, Goncalves AKdS. Perinatal morbidity and mortality associated with chlamydial infection: a meta-analysis study. *Braz J Infect Dis.* 2011;15(6):533-539

Appendix B4. Excluded Studies

Exclusion code: 3

Silveira MF, Ghanem KG, Erbelding EJ, et al. Chlamydia trachomatis infection during pregnancy and the risk of preterm birth: a case-control study. *Int J STD AIDS.* 2009;20(7):465-469
Exclusion code: 4

Singh D, Fine DN, Marrazzo JM. Chlamydia trachomatis infection among women reporting sexual activity with women screened in Family Planning Clinics in the Pacific Northwest, 1997 to 2005. *Am J Public Health.* 2011;101(7):1284-1290
Exclusion code: 5

Sirmatel F, Sahin N, Sirmatel O, Telli E, Kececi S. Chlamydia trachomatis antigen positivity in women in risk groups and its relationship with the use of antibiotics. *Jpn J Infect Dis.* 2005;58(1):41-43
Exclusion code: 4

Skidmore S, Horner P, Herring A, et al. Vulvovaginal-swab or first-catch urine specimen to detect Chlamydia trachomatis in women in a community setting? *J Clin Microbiol.* 2006;44(12):4389-4394
Exclusion code: 3

Skjeldestad FE, Marsico MA, Sings HL, Nordbo SA, Storvold G. Incidence and risk factors for genital Chlamydia trachomatis infection: a 4-year prospective cohort study. *Sex Transm Dis.* 2009;36(5):273-279
Exclusion code: 5

Skovgaard S, Larsen HK, Sand C, et al. Genital and extra-genital screening for gonorrhoea using the BD Probetec ET system with an in-house PCR method targeting the porA pseudogene as confirmatory test. *Acta Derm Venereol.* 2012;92(1):45-49
Exclusion code: 3

Sparrow M, Lewis H, Brown P, Bromhead C, Fernando D, Maitra A. Chlamydia screening in Wellington Family Planning Association (FPA) clinics: a demonstration project. *N Z Med J.* 2007;120(1252):U2490
Exclusion code: 3

Spaulding AC, Clarke JG, Jongco AM, Flanigan TP. Small reservoirs: jail screening for gonorrhea and Chlamydia in low prevalence areas. *J.* 2009;15(1):28-34; quiz 80-21
Exclusion code: 10

Spauwen LWL, Hoebe CJPA, Brouwers EEHG, Dukers-Muijrers NHTM. Improving STD testing behavior among high-risk young adults by offering STD testing at a vocational school. *BMC Public Health.* 2011;11:750
Exclusion code: 10

Spence D. Bad medicine: chlamydia. *BMJ.* 2010;340:c2547
Exclusion code: 7

Spigarelli MG. Urine gonococcal/Chlamydia testing in adolescents. *Curr Opin Obstet Gynecol.* 2006;18(5):498-502
Exclusion code: 6

Stampler KM, Lieberman A, Fraga M, Cohen A, Herman A. Vaginal wet mounts on asymptomatic adolescent females; are they beneficial? *J Pediatr Adolesc Gynecol.* 2008;21(4):227-230
Exclusion code: 4

Stanley B, Todd A. Testing for Neisseria gonorrhoeae by nucleic acid amplification testing of chlamydia samples using Roche Cobas Amplicor in a rural area in the north of England does not find more gonorrhoea in primary care. *Sex Transm Infect.* 2005;81(6):518
Exclusion code: 7

Stary A, Najim B, Lee HH. Vulval swabs as alternative specimens for ligase chain reaction detection of genital chlamydial infection in women. *J Clin Microbiol.* 1997;35(4):836-838
Exclusion code: 4

Stefanski P, Hafner JW, Riley SL, Sunga KLY, Schaefer TJ. Diagnostic utility of the genital Gram stain in ED patients. *Am J Emerg Med.* 2010;28(1):13-18
Exclusion code: 3

Stein CR, Kaufman JS, Ford CA, Leone PA, Feldblum PJ, Miller WC. Screening young adults for prevalent chlamydial infection in community settings. *Ann Epidemiol.* 2008;18(7):560-571
Exclusion code: 3

Stenqvist K, Lindqvist A, Almerson P, Jonsson L, Lander R. [Chlamydia test via Internet a good alternative to testing in clinics]. *Lakartidningen.* 2010;107(6):350-353
Exclusion code: 8

Stephens RS. The cellular paradigm of chlamydial pathogenesis. *Trends Microbiol.* 2003;11(1):44-51

Appendix B4. Excluded Studies

Exclusion code: 2

Stevens MP, Twin J, Fairley CK, et al. Development and evaluation of an ompA quantitative real-time PCR assay for Chlamydia trachomatis serovar determination. *J Clin Microbiol.* 2010;48(6):2060-2065
Exclusion code: 4

Stewart R. Opportunistic chlamydia testing: improving nursing practice through self-audit and reflection. *Nurs Prax N Z.* 2005;21(1):43-52
Exclusion code: 7

Stolte IG, de Wit JBF, Kolader M, Fennema H, Coutinho RA, Dukers NHTM. Association between 'safer sex fatigue' and rectal gonorrhea is mediated by unsafe sex with casual partners among HIV-positive homosexual men. *Sex Transm Dis.* 2006;33(4):201-208
Exclusion code: 5

Storm M, Gustafsson I, Herrmann B, Engstrand L. Real-time PCR for pharmacodynamic studies of Chlamydia trachomatis. *J Microbiol Methods.* 2005;61(3):361-367
Exclusion code: 3

Stuart B, Hinde A. Identifying individuals engaging in risky sexual behaviour for chlamydia infection in the UK: a latent class approach. *J Biosoc Sci.* 2010;42(1):27-42
Exclusion code: 5

Sturm PDJ, Connolly C, Khan N, Ebrahim S, Sturm AW. Vaginal tampons as specimen collection device for the molecular diagnosis of non-ulcerative sexually transmitted infections in antenatal clinic attendees. *Int J STD AIDS.* 2004;15(2):94-98
Exclusion code: 3

Su W-H, Tsou T-S, Chen C-S, et al. Are we satisfied with the tools for the diagnosis of gonococcal infection in females? *J Chin Med Assoc.* 2011;74(10):430-434
Exclusion code: 7

Su W-H, Tsou T-S, Chen C-S, et al. Diagnosis of Chlamydia infection in women. *Taiwan.* 2011;50(3):261-267
Exclusion code: 12

Sufrin CB, Postlethwaite D, Armstrong MA, Merchant M, Wendt JM, Steinauer JE. Neisseria gonorrhea and Chlamydia trachomatis screening at

intrauterine device insertion and pelvic inflammatory disease. *Obstet Gynecol.* 2012;120(6):1314-1321
Exclusion code: 5

Sullivan EA, Abel M, Tabrizi S, et al. Prevalence of sexually transmitted infections among antenatal women in Vanuatu, 1999-2000. *Sex Transm Dis.* 2003;30(4):362-366
Exclusion code: 5

Suzuki K, Matsumoto T, Murakami H, Tateda K, Ishii N, Yamaguchi K. Evaluation of a rapid antigen detection test for Neisseria gonorrhoeae in urine sediment for diagnosis of gonococcal urethritis in males. *J Infect Chemother.* 2004;10(4):208-211
Exclusion code: 4

Svenstrup HF, Fedder J, Kristoffersen SE, Trolle B, Birkelund S, Christiansen G. Mycoplasma genitalium, Chlamydia trachomatis, and tubal factor infertility--a prospective study. *Fertil Steril.* 2008;90(3):513-520
Exclusion code: 3

Swain GR, McDonald RA, Pfister JR, Gradus MS, Sedmak GV, Singh A. Decision analysis: point-of-care Chlamydia testing vs. laboratory-based methods. *Clin.* 2004;2(1):29-35
Exclusion code: 3

Swedish Council on Health Technology Assessment. Urine Specimens in Diagnosing Chlamydia in Women. *SBU Alert.* Vol 052010
Exclusion code: 4

Tabrizi S, Chen S, Fairley C, et al. Tampon-collected genital cells in the detection of Chlamydia trachomatis by polymerase chain reaction. *J Infect Dis.* 1993;168(3):796-797
Exclusion code: 4

Tabrizi SN, Chen S, Tapsall J, Garland SM. Evaluation of opa-based real-time PCR for detection of Neisseria gonorrhoeae. *Sex Transm Dis.* 2005;32(3):199-202
Exclusion code: 4

Tabrizi SN, Fairley CK, Cehn S, et al. Evaluation of patient-administered tampon specimens for Chlamydia trachomatis and Neisseria gonorrhoeae. *Sex Transm Dis.* 2000;27(3):133-137
Exclusion code: 4

Tabrizi SN, Paterson B, Fairley CK, Bowden FJ, Garland SM. A self-administered technique for the

detection of sexually transmitted diseases in remote communities. *J Infect Dis.* 1997;176(1):289-292
Exclusion code: 3

Tabrizi SN, Paterson BA, Fairley CK, Bowden FJ, Garland SM. Comparison of tampon and urine as self-administered methods of specimen collection in the detection of Chlamydia trachomatis, Neisseria gonorrhoeae and Trichomonas vaginalis in women. *Int J STD AIDS.* 1998;9(6):347-349
Exclusion code: 4

Tabrizi SN, Skov S, Chandeying V, Norpech J, Garland SM. Prevalence of sexually transmitted infections among clients of female commercial sex workers in Thailand. *Sex Transm Dis.* 2000;27(6):358-362
Exclusion code: 10

Taha NSA, Focchi J, Ribalta JCL, Castelo A, Lorincz A, Dores GB. Universal Collection Medium (UCM) is as suitable as the Standard Transport Medium (STM) for Hybrid Capture II (HC-2) assay. *J Clin Virol.* 2006;36(1):32-35
Exclusion code: 4

Tang J, Xu Z, Zhou L, Qin H, Wang Y, Wang H. Rapid and simultaneous detection of Ureaplasma parvum and Chlamydia trachomatis antibodies based on visual protein microarray using gold nanoparticles and silver enhancement. *Diagn Microbiol Infect Dis.* 2010;67(2):122-128
Exclusion code: 5

Tao G, Hoover KW, Kent CK. Chlamydia testing patterns for commercially insured women, 2008. *Am J Prev Med.* 2012;42(4):337-341
Exclusion code: 5

Tao G, Irwin KL. Receipt of HIV and STD testing services during routine general medical or gynecological examinations: Variations by patient sexual risk behaviors. *Sex Transm Dis.* 2008;35(2):167-171
Exclusion code: 2

Tao G, Tian LH, Peterman TA. Estimating Chlamydia screening rates by using reported sexually transmitted disease tests for sexually active women aged 16 to 25 years in the United States. *Sex Transm Dis.* 2007;34(3):180-182
Exclusion code: 5

Tebb K, Wibbelsman C, Ko T, Neuhaus JM, Shafer M-A. Translating and sustaining a chlamydial

screening intervention 4 years later. *Arch Intern Med.* 2011;171(19):1767-1768
Exclusion code: 5

Tebb KP, Pantell RH, Wibbelsman CJ, et al. Screening sexually active adolescents for Chlamydia trachomatis: what about the boys? *Am J Public Health.* 2005;95(10):1806-1810
Exclusion code: 5

Tebb KP, Wibbelsman C, Neuhaus JM, Shafer M-A. Screening for asymptomatic Chlamydia infections among sexually active adolescent girls during pediatric urgent care. *Arch Pediatr Adolesc Med.* 2009;163(6):559-564
Exclusion code: 5

Templeton DJ, Jin F, Imrie J, et al. Prevalence, incidence and risk factors for pharyngeal chlamydia in the community based Health in Men (HIM) cohort of homosexual men in Sydney, Australia. *Sex Transm Infect.* 2008;84(5):361-363
Exclusion code: 5

Templeton DJ, Manokaran N, O'Connor CC. Prevalence and predictors of chlamydia co-infection among patients infected with gonorrhoea at a sexual health clinic in Sydney. *Sex Health.* 2012;9(4):392-394
Exclusion code: 5

Templeton DJ, Wang Y, Higgins AN, Manokaran N. Self-collected anal swabs in men who have sex with men: minimal benefit of routine peri-anal examination. *Sex Transm Infect.* 2011;87(3):204
Exclusion code: 10

Thomas G, Humphris G, Ozakinci G, et al. A qualitative study of pharmacists' views on offering chlamydia screening to women requesting Emergency Hormonal Contraception. *Bjog.* 2010;117(1):109-113
Exclusion code: 5

Thomas TL, Nandram B. Predicting incidence and asymptomatic rates for chlamydia in small domains. *J Adv Nurs.* 2010;66(12):2650-2658
Exclusion code: 5

Tikkanen M, Surcel HM, Bloigu A, et al. Prediction of placental abruption by testing for C-reactive protein and chlamydial antibody levels in early pregnancy. *Bjog.* 2008;115(4):486-491
Exclusion code: 4

Appendix B4. Excluded Studies

Tinmouth J, Gilmour MW, Kovacs C, et al. Is there a reservoir of sub-clinical lymphogranuloma venereum and non-LGV Chlamydia trachomatis infection in men who have sex with men? *Int J STD AIDS.* 2008;19(12):805-809
Exclusion code: 5

Tipple C, Hill SC, Smith A. Is screening for pharyngeal Chlamydia trachomatis warranted in high-risk groups? *Int J STD AIDS.* 2010;21(11):770-771
Exclusion code: 4

Tomanovic S, Cukic I, Obradovic M, Curcic N, Petrovic-Milinkovic A, Djukic S. [The diagnosis of Chlamydia trachomatis cervical infection among students by using classical and molecular methods]. *Srp Arh Celok Lek.* 2013;141(3-4):187-191
Exclusion code: 8

Tomanovic S, Dukic S. [Classical and molecular methods for diagnosis of Chlamydia trachomatis infections]. *Med Pregl.* 2011;64(9-10):477-480
Exclusion code: 7

Toro MC. Closing in on Chlamydia. *Nursing.* 2008;38(9):61
Exclusion code: 7

Tosun I, Cihanyurdu M, Kaklikkaya N, Topbas M, Aydin F, Erturk M. Asymptomatic Chlamydia trachomatis infection and predictive criteria among low-risk women in a primary care setting. *Jpn J Infect Dis.* 2008,61(3):216-218
Exclusion code: 5

Toth M, Patton DL, Esquenazi B, Shevchuk M, Thaler H, Divon M. Association between Chlamydia trachomatis and abnormal uterine bleeding. *Am J Reprod Immunol.* 2007;57(5):361-366
Exclusion code: 4

Tran K, Nkansah E. Urine based testing for Gonorrhea and Chlamydia: A review of diagnostic accuracy, cost-effectiveness, and compliance. Health Technology Inquiry Service 2009.
Exclusion code: 12

Tran K, Nkansah E. Urine based testing for gonorrhea and chlamydia: a review of diagnostic accuracy, cost-effectiveness, and compliance (Structured abstract). *Health Technology Assessment Database.* 2013(1)
Exclusion code: 2

Tsesliuk MV, Gushchin AE, Savochkina IA, Bykov AS, Shipulin GA. [Comparison of methods for laboratory diagnosis of Neisseria gonorrhoeae by using the "extended gold standard"]. *Klin Lab Diagn.* 2008(7):48-52
Exclusion code: 8

Tsuruoka N, Uzawa Y, Kikuchi K, Ohtsuka H, Todome Y, Ohkuni H. [Evaluation of the GonoGen II kit for rapid identification of Neisseria gonorrhoeae using monoclonal antibody directed at gonococcal outer membrane protein 1]. *Kansenshogaku Zasshi.* 2008;82(4):317-321
Exclusion code: 8

U.S. Preventive Services Task Force. Screening for Gonorrhea: Recommendation Statement. *American Academy of Family Physicians.* 2005;3(3):263-267
Exclusion code: 2

U.S. Preventive Services Task Force. Procedure Manual. 2011; U.S. Preventive Services Task Force. Rockvile, MD. Available at: http://www.uspreventiveservicestaskforce.org/uspstf08/methods/procmanual.htm. Accessed 15 April, 2014
Exclusion code: 2.

U.S. Preventive Services Task Force, Calonge N, Petitti DB, et al. Screening for chlamydial infection: U.S. Preventive Services Task Force recommendation statement. *Ann Intern Med.* 2007;147(2):128-134
Exclusion code: 2

Uuskula A, Kals M, McNutt L-A. Assessing non-response to a mailed health survey including self-collection of biological material. *Eur J Public Health.* 2011;21(4):538-542
Exclusion code: 5

van Bergen J. Chlamydia infection. Screening needs more answers. *BMJ.* 2010;340:c2502
Exclusion code: 7

van Bergen JEAM, Fennema JSA, van den Broek IVF, et al. Rationale, design, and results of the first screening round of a comprehensive, register-based, Chlamydia screening implementation programme in the Netherlands. *BMC Infect Dis.* 2010;10:293
Exclusion code: 2

van den Bos RR, van der Meijden WI. Persistent high-risk sexual behaviour in men who have sex with men after symptomatic lymphogranuloma venereum proctitis. *Int J STD AIDS.* 2007;18(10):715-716
Exclusion code: 3

Appendix B4. Excluded Studies

van den Broek IVF, Brouwers EEHG, Gotz HM, et al. Systematic selection of screening participants by risk score in a Chlamydia screening programme is feasible and effective. *Sex Transm Infect.* 2012;88(3):205-211
Exclusion code: 5

van den Broek IVF, Hoebe CJPA, van Bergen JEAM, et al. Evaluation design of a systematic, selective, internet-based, Chlamydia screening implementation in the Netherlands, 2008-2010: implications of first results for the analysis. *BMC Infect Dis.* 2010;10:89
Exclusion code: 3

van den Broek IVF, van Bergen JEAM, Brouwers EEHG, et al. Effectiveness of yearly, register based screening for chlamydia in the Netherlands: controlled trial with randomised stepped wedge implementation. *BMJ.* 2012;345:e4316
Exclusion code: 5

Van der Bij AK, Spaargaren J, Morre SA, et al. Diagnostic and clinical implications of anorectal lymphogranuloma venereum in men who have sex with men: a retrospective case-control study. *Clin Infect Dis.* 2006;42(2):186-194
Exclusion code: 5

van der Helm JJ, Hoebe CJPA, van Rooijen MS, et al. High performance and acceptability of self-collected rectal swabs for diagnosis of Chlamydia trachomatis and Neisseria gonorrhoeae in men who have sex with men and women. *Sex Transm Dis.* 2009;36(8):493-497
Exclusion code: 4

van der Helm JJ, Sabajo LOA, Grunberg AW, Morre SA, Speksnijder AGCL, de Vries HJC. Point-of-care test for detection of urogenital chlamydia in women shows low sensitivity. A performance evaluation study in two clinics in Suriname. *PLoS ONE.* 2012;7(2):e32122
Exclusion code: 3

Van Der Pol B, Kraft CS, Williams JA. Use of an adaptation of a commercially available PCR assay aimed at diagnosis of chlamydia and gonorrhea to detect Trichomonas vaginalis in urogenital specimens. *J Clin Microbiol.* 2006;44(2):366-373
Exclusion code: 5

Van Der Pol B, Taylor SN, Liesenfeld O, Williams JA, Hook EW, 3rd. Vaginal swabs are the optimal specimen for detection of genital Chlamydia trachomatis or Neisseria gonorrhoeae using the Cobas 4800 CT/NG test. *Sex Transm Dis.* 2013;40(3):247-250
Exclusion code: 3

van Dommelen L, Dukers-Muijrers N, van Tiel FH, Brouwers EEHG, Hoebe CJPA. Evaluation of one-sample testing of self-obtained vaginal swabs and first catch urine samples separately and in combination for the detection of Chlamydia trachomatis by two amplified DNA assays in women visiting a sexually transmitted disease clinic. *Sex Transm Dis.* 2011;38(6):533-535
Exclusion code: 3

van Dommelen L, van Tiel FH, Ouburg S, et al. Alarmingly poor performance in Chlamydia trachomatis point-of-care testing. *Sex Transm Infect.* 2010;86(5):355-359
Exclusion code: 4

Van Dyck E, Ieven M, Pattyn S, Van Damme L, Laga M. Detection of Chlamydia trachomatis and Neisseria gonorrhoeae by enzyme immunoassay, culture, and three nucleic acid amplification tests. *J Clin Microbiol.* 2001;39(5):1751-1756
Exclusion code: 3

Vaughan D, O'Connell E, Cormican M, et al. "Pee-in-a-Pot": acceptability and uptake of on-site chlamydia screening in a student population in the Republic of Ireland. *BMC Infect Dis.* 2010;10:325
Exclusion code: 5

Venkatesh KK, van der Straten A, Cheng H, et al. The relative contribution of viral and bacterial sexually transmitted infections on HIV acquisition in southern African women in the Methods for Improving Reproductive Health in Africa study. *Int J STD AIDS.* 2011;22(4):218-224
Exclusion code: 4

Verhelst R, Verstraelen H, Claeys G, et al. Comparison between Gram stain and culture for the characterization of vaginal microflora: definition of a distinct grade that resembles grade I microflora and revised categorization of grade I microflora. *BMC Microbiol.* 2005;5:61
Exclusion code: 3

Verhoeven V, Avonts D, Van Royen P, Denekens J. Implementation of a pilot programme for screening for chlamydial infection in general practice. *Eur J Gen Pract.* 2004;10(4):157-161
Exclusion code: 3

Appendix B4. Excluded Studies

Verhoeven V, Avonts D, Van Royen P, Weyler J, Wang X, Stalpaert M. Performance of a screening algorithm for chlamydial infection in 2 samples of patients in general practice. *Scand J Infect Dis.* 2004;36(11-12):873-875
Exclusion code: 3

Verhoeven V, Baay M, Weyler J, et al. Concomitant Chlamydia trachomatis and human papilloma virus infection cannot be attributed solely to sexual behaviour. *Eur J Clin Microbiol Infect Dis.* 2004;23(9):735-737
Exclusion code: 5

Verkooyen RP, Noordhoek GT, Klapper PE, et al. Reliability of nucleic acid amplification methods for detection of Chlamydia trachomatis in urine: results of the first international collaborative quality control study among 96 laboratories. *J Clin Microbiol.* 2003;41(7):3013-3016
Exclusion code: 4

Verma R, Sood S, Bala M, et al. Diagnostic implications of 16S ribosomal assay for gonorrhoea. *Sex Transm Infect.* 2010;86(6):461-464
Exclusion code: 4

Verma R, Sood S, Bala M, et al. Evaluation of an opa gene-based nucleic acid amplification test for detection of Neisseria gonorrhoeae in urogenital samples in North India. *Epidemiol Infect.* 2012;140(11):2110-2116
Exclusion code: 4

Vernel-Pauillac F, Merien F. A novel real-time duplex PCR assay for detecting penA and ponA genotypes in Neisseria gonorrhoeae: Comparison with phenotypes determined by the E-test. *Clin Chem.* 2006;52(12):2294-2296
Exclusion code: 4

Vickerman P, Watts C, Alary M, Mabey D, Peeling RW. Sensitivity requirements for the point of care diagnosis of Chlamydia trachomatis and Neisseria gonorrhocae in women. *Sex Transm Infect.* 2003;79(5):363-367
Exclusion code: 5

Voelker R. Experts reconsider wisdom of limiting Chlamydia screening only to women. *Jama.* 2010;303(9):823-824
Exclusion code: 7

Walker J, Fairley CK, Walker SM, et al. Computer reminders for Chlamydia screening in general practice: a randomized controlled trial. *Sex Transm Dis.* 2010;37(7):445-450
Exclusion code: 4

Wallace LA, Scoular A, Hart G, Reid M, Wilson P, Goldberg DJ. What is the excess risk of infertility in women after genital chlamydia infection? A systematic review of the evidence. *Sex Transm Infect.* 2008;84(3):171-175
Exclusion code: 3

Wallin KL, Wiklund F, Luostarinen T, et al. A population-based prospective study of Chlamydia trachomatis infection and cervical carcinoma. *Int J Cancer.* 2002;101(4):371-374
Exclusion code: 2

Walsh A, Rourke FO, Crowley B. Molecular detection and confirmation of Neisseria gonorrhoeae in urogenital and extragenital specimens using the Abbott CT/NG RealTime assay and an in-house assay targeting the porA pseudogene. *Eur J Clin Microbiol Infect Dis.* 2011;30(4):561-567
Exclusion code: 3

Walsh A, Rourke FO, Laoi BN, Crowley B. Evaluation of the Abbott RealTime CT assay with the BD ProbeTec ET assay for the detection of Chlamydia trachomatis in a clinical microbiology laboratory. *Diagn Microbiol Infect Dis.* 2009;64(1):13-19
Exclusion code: 3

Wand H, Ramjee G. The effects of injectable hormonal contraceptives on HIV seroconversion and on sexually transmitted infections. *Aids.* 2012;26(3):375-380
Exclusion code: 5

Watchirs Smith LA, Hillman R, Ward J, et al. Point-of-care tests for the diagnosis of Neisseria gonorrhoeae infection: a systematic review of operational and performance characteristics. *Sex Transm Infect.* 2013;89(4):320-326
Exclusion code: 4

Watson EJ, Templeton A, Russell I, et al. The accuracy and efficacy of screening tests for Chlamydia trachomatis: a systematic review. *J Med Microbiol.* 2002;51(12):1021-1031
Exclusion code: 12

Watson V, Ryan M, Watson E. Valuing experience factors in the provision of Chlamydia screening: an application to women attending the family planning clinic. *Value Health.* 2009;12(4):621-623

Appendix B4. Excluded Studies

Exclusion code: 5

Webber MP, Schoenbaum EE, Farzadegan H, Klein RS. Tampons as a self-administered collection method for the detection and quantification of genital HIV-1. *Aids.* 2001;15(11):1417-1420
Exclusion code: 5

Webley WC, Tilahun Y, Lay K, et al. Occurrence of Chlamydia trachomatis and Chlamydia pneumoniae in paediatric respiratory infections. *Eur Respir J.* 2009;33(2):360-367
Exclusion code: 5

Weissenbacher TM, Kupka MS, Kainer F, Friese K, Mylonas I. Screening for Chlamydia trachomatis in pregnancy: a retrospective analysis in a German urban area. *Arch Gynecol Obstet.* 2011;283(6):1343-1347
Exclusion code: 5

Weisz J, Lozyniak S, Lane SD, et al. It takes at least two: male partner factors, racial/ethnic disparity, and Chlamydia trachomatis among pregnant women. *J Health Care Poor Underserved.* 2011;22(3):871-885
Exclusion code: 5

West ES, Munoz B, Mkocha H, et al. Mass treatment and the effect on the load of Chlamydia trachomatis infection in a trachoma-hyperendemic community. *Invest Ophthalmol Vis Sci.* 2005;46(1):83-87
Exclusion code: 4

Wheeler HL, Skinner CJ, Khunda A, Aitken C, Perpanthan D, Staite E. Molecular testing (strand displacement assay) for identification of urethral gonorrhoea in men: can it replace culture as the gold standard? *Int J STD AIDS.* 2005;16(6):430-432
Exclusion code: 3

Whiley DM, Buda PJ, Bayliss J, Cover L, Bates J, Sloots TP. A new confirmatory Neisseria gonorrhoeae real-time PCR assay targeting the porA pseudogene. *Eur J Clin Microbiol Infect Dis.* 2004;23(9):705-710
Exclusion code: 3

Whiley DM, Buda PP, Freeman K, Pattle NI, Bates J, Sloots TP. A real-time PCR assay for the detection of Neisseria gonorrhoeae in genital and extragenital specimens. *Diagn Microbiol Infect Dis.* 2005;52(1):1-5
Exclusion code: 3

Whiley DM, Goire N, Ray ES, et al. Neisseria gonorrhoeae multi-antigen sequence typing using non-cultured clinical specimens. *Sex Transm Infect.* 2010;86(1):51-55
Exclusion code: 3

Whiley DM, Sloots TP. Comparison of three in-house multiplex PCR assays for the detection of Neisseria gonorrhoeae and Chlamydia trachomatis using real-time and conventional detection methodologies. *Pathology.* 2005;37(5):364-370
Exclusion code: 4

Whiley DM, Tapsall JW, Sloots TP. Nucleic acid amplification testing for Neisseria gonorrhoeae: an ongoing challenge. *J Mol Diagn.* 2006;8(1):3-15
Exclusion code: 7

Wiehe SE, Rosenman MB, Wang J, Fortenberry JD. Disparities in chlamydia testing among young women with sexually transmitted infection symptoms. *Sex Transm Dis.* 2010;37(12):751-755
Exclusion code: 2

Wiehe SE, Rosenman MB, Wang J, Katz BP, Fortenberry JD. Chlamydia screening among young women: individual- and provider-level differences in testing. *Pediatrics.* 2011;127(2):e336-344
Exclusion code: 5

Wiesenfeld HC, Heine RP, Rideout A, Macio I, DiBiasi F, Sweet RL. The vaginal introitus: a novel site for Chlamydia trachomatis testing in women. *Am J Obstet Gynecol.* 1996;174(5):1542-1546
Exclusion code: 3

Wilkinson A, El-Hayek C, Fairley CK, et al. Incidence and risk factors associated with chlamydia in men who have sex with men: a cohort analysis of Victorian Primary Care Network for Sentinel Surveillance data. *Sex Transm Infect.* 2012;88(5):319-324
Exclusion code: 5

Wilkowska-Trojniel M, Zdrodowska-Stefanow B, Ostaszewska-Puchalska I, Redzko S, Przepiesc J, Zdrodowski M. The influence of Chlamydia trachomatis infection on spontaneous abortions. *Adv Med Sci.* 2009;54(1):86-90
Exclusion code: 5

Wills GS, Horner PJ, Reynolds R, et al. Pgp3 antibody enzyme-linked immunosorbent assay, a sensitive and specific assay for seroepidemiological analysis of Chlamydia trachomatis infection. *Clin Vaccine Immunol.* 2009;16(6):835-843
Exclusion code: 3

Appendix B4. Excluded Studies

Winscott M, Taylor M, Kenney K. Sexually transmitted diseases among American Indians in Arizona: an important public health disparity. *Public Health Rep.* 2010;125 Suppl 4:51-60
Exclusion code: 5

Wong A, Maclean AB, Furrows SJ, Ridgway GL, Hardiman PJ, Perrett CW. Could epithelial ovarian cancer be associated with chlamydial infection? *Eur J Gynaecol Oncol.* 2007;28(2):117-120
Exclusion code: 5

Wood BJ, Gaydos JC, McKee KT, Jr., Gaydos CA. Comparison of the urine Leukocyte Esterase Test to a Nucleic Acid Amplification Test for screening non-health care-seeking male soldiers for Chlamydia trachomatis and Neisseria gonorrhoeae infections. *Mil Med.* 2007;172(7):770-772
Exclusion code: 4

Workowski KA, Berman S. Sexually transmitted diseases treatment guidelines, 2010. *MMWR Recomm Rep.* 2010;59(12 RR):1-113
Exclusion code: 2

Wozniakowska-Gesicka T, Wisniewska-Ligier M, Kicinski P, Gesicki T. [Underestimated problem of Chlamydia infections]. *Przegl Epidemiol.* 2008;62 Suppl 1:133-141
Exclusion code: 8

Wright TC, Jr., Denny L, Kuhn L, Pollack A, Lorincz A. HPV DNA testing of self-collected vaginal samples compared with cytologic screening to detect cervical cancer. *Jama.* 2000;283(1):81-86
Exclusion code: 5

Xia Q-F, Xu S-X, Wang D-S, et al. Development of a novel quantitative real-time assay using duplex scorpion primer for detection of Chlamydia trachomatis. *Exp Mol Pathol.* 2007;83(1):119-124
Exclusion code: 4

Xiong L, Kong F, Zhou H, Gilbert GL. Use of PCR and reverse line blot hybridization assay for rapid simultaneous detection and serovar identification of Chlamydia trachomatis. *J Clin Microbiol.* 2006;44(4):1413-1418
Exclusion code: 4

Xu F, Stoner BP, Taylor SN, et al. Use of home-obtained vaginal swabs to facilitate rescreening for Chlamydia trachomatis infections: two randomized controlled trials. *Obstet Gynecol.* 2011;118(2 Pt 1):231-239
Exclusion code: 3

Yang JL, Schachter J, Moncada J, et al. Comparison of an rRNA-based and DNA-based nucleic acid amplification test for the detection of Chlamydia trachomatis in trachoma. *Br J Ophthalmol.* 2007;91(3):293-295
Exclusion code: 3

Yang J-M, Liu H-X, Hao Y-X, He C, Zhao D-M. Development of a rapid real-time PCR assay for detection and quantification of four familiar species of Chlamydiaceae. *J Clin Virol.* 2006;36(1):79-81
Exclusion code: 4

Yeung A, Bush M, Cummings R, et al. Use of computerized medical records to determine the feasibility of testing for chlamydia without patients seeing a practitioner. *Int J STD AIDS.* 2010;21(11):755-757
Exclusion code: 4

Yip P-p, Chan W-h, Yip K-t, Que T-l, Kwong N-s, Ho C-k. The use of polymerase chain reaction assay versus conventional methods in detecting neonatal chlamydial conjunctivitis. *J Pediatr Ophthalmol Strabismus.* 2008;45(4):234-239
Exclusion code: 3

Young F. Sexually transmitted infections. Genital chlamydia: practical management in primary care. *J Fam Health Care.* 2005;15(1):19-21
Exclusion code: 7

Young H, Anderson J, Moyes A, McMillan A. Non-cultural detection of rectal and pharyngeal gonorrhoea by the Gen-Probe PACE 2 assay. *Genitourin Med.* 1997;73(1):59-62
Exclusion code: 2

Zampini AN. Emergency prevention: the benefit of chlamydia and gonorrhea screening in urban emergency departments. *J Emerg Nurs.* 2010;36(3):246-247
Exclusion code: 7

Zbroch T, Knapp P, Blonska E, Kobylec M, Knapp P. [Life style, Chlamydia trachomatis infection, bacterial vaginosis and their impact on the frequency of cervical lesions]. *Ginekol Pol.* 2004;75(7):538-544
Exclusion code: 8

Zenner D, Molinar D, Nichols T, Riha J, Macintosh M, Nardone A. Should young people be paid for getting tested? A national comparative study to evaluate patient financial incentives for chlamydia screening. *BMC Public Health.* 2012;12:261
Exclusion code: 5

Appendix B4. Excluded Studies

Zhang L-d, Pei J, Zhang H-m, Sun X-f. [Relationship between mycoplasma and chlamydia infection and lesions in the cervical tissue in high-risk HPV-positive patients]. *Chung Hua Shih Yen Ho Lin Chuang Ping Tu Hsueh.* 2010;24(5):346-348
Exclusion code: 8

Zheng H-p, Jiang L-f, Fang D-y, et al. Application of an oligonucleotide array assay for rapid detecting and genotyping of Chlamydia trachomatis from urogenital specimens. *Diagn Microbiol Infect Dis.* 2007;57(1):1-6
Exclusion code: 4

Zhong X-Y, Yu J-L, Wang J, et al. [Genotyping of major outer membrane protein gene of Chlamydia trachomatis by cleavase fragment length polymorphism analysis]. *Zhonghua Er Ke Za Zhi.* 2005;43(1):5-8
Exclusion code: 8

Zou H, Fairley CK, Guy R, Chen MY. The efficacy of clinic-based interventions aimed at increasing screening for bacterial sexually transmitted infections among men who have sex with men: a systematic review. *Sex Transm Dis.* 2012;39(5):382-387
Exclusion code: 4

Appendix B5. Quality Rating Criteria

Randomized, Controlled Trials (RCTs) and Cohort Studies

Criteria:

- Initial assembly of comparable groups:
  - for RCTs: adequate randomization, including first concealment and whether potential confounders were distributed equally among groups
  - for cohort studies: consideration of potential confounders with either restriction or measurement for adjustment in the analysis; consideration of inception cohorts
- Maintenance of comparable groups (includes attrition, crossovers, adherence, contamination)
- Important differential loss to followup or overall high loss to followup
- Measurements: equal, reliable, and valid (includes masking of outcome assessment)
- Clear definition of interventions
- Important outcomes considered
- Analysis: adjustment for potential confounders for cohort studies, or intention-to-treat analysis for RCTs.

Definition of ratings based on above criteria:

Good: Meets all criteria: Comparable groups are assembled initially and maintained throughout the study (followup at least 80%); reliable and valid measurement instruments are used and applied equally to the groups; interventions are spelled out clearly; important outcomes are considered; and appropriate attention to confounders in analysis. In addition, for RCTs, intention to treat analysis is used.

Fair: Studies will be graded "fair" if any or all of the following problems occur, without the fatal flaws noted in the "poor" category below: Generally comparable groups are assembled initially but some question remains whether some (although not major) differences occurred in follow-up; measurement instruments are acceptable (although not the best) and generally applied equally; some but not all important outcomes are considered; and some but not all potential confounders are accounted for. Intention to treat analysis is done for RCTs.

Poor: Studies will be graded "poor" if any of the following fatal flaws exists: Groups assembled initially are not close to being comparable or maintained throughout the study; unreliable or invalid measurement instruments are used or not applied at all equally among groups (including not masking outcome assessment); and key confounders are given little or no attention. For RCTs, intention to treat is lacking.

Diagnostic Accuracy Studies

Criteria:

- Screening test relevant, available for primary care, adequately described
- Study uses a credible reference standard, performed regardless of test results
- Reference standard interpreted independently of screening test
- Handles indeterminate results in a reasonable manner
- Spectrum of patients included in study
- Sample size
- Administration of reliable screening test

Definition of ratings based on above criteria:

Good: Evaluates relevant available screening test; uses a credible reference standard; interprets reference standard independently of screening test; reliability of test assessed; has few or handles indeterminate results in a reasonable manner; includes large number (more than 100) broad-spectrum patients with and without disease.

Fair: Evaluates relevant available screening test; uses reasonable although not best standard; interprets reference standard independent of screening test; moderate sample size (50 to 100 subjects) and a "medium" spectrum of patients.

Poor: Has fatal flaw such as: uses inappropriate reference standard; screening test improperly administered; biased ascertainment of reference standard; very small sample size of very narrow selected spectrum of patients.

Source: USPSTF Procedure Manual[24]

Heidi Bauer, MD, MS, MPH
Chief, Sexually Transmitted Disease, Control Branch, California Department of Public Health, CA; Adjunct Assistant Professor, Department of Epidemiology and Biostatistics, Division of Preventive Medicine and Public Health, University of California San Francisco, San Francisco, CA; Assistant Adjunct Professor, Division of Epidemiology, University of California Berkeley, Berkeley, CA

David D. Celentano, ScD, MHS
Professor, Charles Armstrong Chair, Department of Epidemiology, Johns Hopkins Bloomberg School of Public Health, Baltimore, MD

Christopher Fairley, MBBS, PhD
Melbourne Sexual Health Centre, Alfred Hospital, Carlton, Victoria, Australia; Sexual Health Unit, Melbourne School of Population Health, The University of Melbourne, Carlton, Victoria, Australia

Khalil Ghanem, MD, PhD
Johns Hopkins University School of Medicine, Baltimore MD

Pippa Oakeshott, MA, MD
Division of Population Health Sciences, St. George's, University of London, United Kingdom

Stephanie N. Taylor, MD
Professor of Medicine and Microbiology, Section of Infectious Disease, Louisiania State University Health Sciences Center, New Orleans, LA; Clinic Administrator and Medical Director, Delgado Personal Health Center Sexually Transmitted Disease Clinic, New Orleans, LA

Rachel Gorwitz, MD, MPH
Medical Epidemiologist, Centers for Disease Control and Prevention

Sarah Kidd, MD, MPH
Medical Epidemiologist, Centers for Disease Control and Prevention

John Papp, PhD
Team Lead, Chlamydia and Gonorrhea Reference Laboratory, Centers for Disease Control and Prevention

Elizabeth Torrone, MSPH, PhD
Epidemiologist, Centers for Disease Control and Prevention

Appendix C1. Randomized, Controlled Trial of Effectiveness of Screening for Chlamydia

Author, year, title	Population characteristics	Eligibility criteria	Number approached, eligible, enrolled, & analyzed	Country & setting	Duration of followup	Attrition	Interventions	Outcomes	Adverse events/ harms	Sponsor	Quality rating
Oakeshott et al, 2010[26] (with data from personal communication) Prevention of Pelvic Infection (POPI) trial	Age (mean): 20.9 y 100% Female 61.1% White 27.2% Black 3.6% Asian 7.5% Other	Sexually active women age ≤27 y. Excluded those who have never had sexual intercourse, have been tested for chlamydial infection in the past 3 months, or were pregnant.	Approached: 3528 Eligible: 2563 Enrolled: 2529 Analyzed: 2377 (1648 asymptomatic women)	UK General population	1 y	Screened: 5% Deferred: 7%	Immediate screening vs. deferred screening after 1 y	Incidence of PID in asymptomatic women: Screened: 0.6% (5/787) Deferred: 1.6% (14/861) RR, 0.39 (95% CI, 0.14 to 1.08) In all women: Screened: 1.3% (15/1191) Deferred: 1.9% (23/1186) RR, 0.65 (95% CI, 0.34 to 1.22)	Not reported	Grant from the Bupa Foundation	Good

Abbreviations: CI = confidence interval; PID = pelvic inflammatory disease; RR = relative risk; UK = United Kingdom.

Appendix C2. Quality Rating of Randomized, Controlled Trial

Author, Year	Randomization adequate?	Allocation concealment adequate?	Groups similar at baseline?	Eligibility criteria specified?	Outcome assessors masked?	Care provider masked?	Patient masked?	Attrition, crossovers, adherence, and contamination reported?	Loss to followup differential /high?	Patients analyzed in the groups to which they were randomized?	Post-randomization exclusions?	Outcomes pre-specified?	Funding source	External validity	Quality Rating
Oakeshott et al, 2010[26]	Yes	Yes	Yes	Yes	Yes	Screener: Yes Treatment: No	Yes	Yes	No/No	Yes	No	Yes	Grant from the Bupa Foundation	High	Good

Appendix C3. Observational Study of Screening Strategies for Chlamydia

Author, year, title	Study design	Country & setting	Interventions	Study duration Mean followup	Baseline demographics
Gotz et al, 2006[25] "Prediction of *Chlamydia trachomatis* infection: application of a scoring rule to other populations"	Observationa Population-based setting	Amsterdam/ Rotterdam	Self-administered questionnaire to develop a prediction rule for probability of infection in participants A: CT pilot study, 2002 to 2003, n=6303 Validation study B: Amsterdam, 1996 to 1997, n=1788 C: Rotterdam, r=172 (high-risk youth)	1 year	**A, B, C** CT result Neg: 5997 (98%), 1361 (96%), 133 (88%) Pos: 144 (2%), 52 (4%), 19 (13%) Sex F: 4195 (68%), 913 (65%), 91 (60%) M: 1946 (32%), 500 (35%), 61 (40%) Age 15 to 19: 1386 (23%), 118 (8%), 87 (58%) 20 to 24: 2307 (38%), 440 (31%), 51 (34%) 25 to 29: 2448 (40%), 855 (61%), 12 (85%) Urogenital symptoms, women No: 4017 (96%), 870 (95%), 84 (92%) Yes: 178 (4%), 43 (5%), 7 (8%) Urogenital symptoms, men No: 1851 (95%), 480 (96%), 59 (97%) Yes: 95 (5%), 20 (4%), 2 (3%) Lifetime sexual partners 1: 2160 (35%), 248 (18%), 34 (22%) 2 to 5: 2904 (47%), 529 (37%), 66 (43%) ≥6: 1077 (18%), 636 (45%), 52 (34%)

Author, year, title	Eligibility criteria	Number enrolled Number analyzed Withdrawals Loss to followup	Adjusted variables for statistical analysis	Intermediate/clinical health outcome results	Adverse events/ harms	Sponsor	Quality rating
See above	Men and women ages 15 to 40 y; sexually active in the past 6 mo	Eligible: 21,000 Enrolled A: 6303 (41% participation rate) B: 1788 C: 172 Excluded: NR Analyzed A: 6141 B: 1413 C: 152 Withdrawals: NR Lost: NR	Discriminatory score AUC used as a model	Performance of predictor score at development and external validation: AUC* (95% CI) A: 0.79 (0.76 to 0.84) B: 0.66 (0.58 to 0.74) C: 0.68 (0.58 to 0.79) Predicted mean prevalence A: 2.3 B: 4.7 C: 8.9 Actual mean prevalence A: 2.3 B: 3.7 C: 12.5	NR	Rotterdam public health service	Good

* Results reflect higher homogeneity in risk factors.
Note: a model with an AUC of 0.5 has no discriminative power, whereas an AUC of 1 reflects perfect discrimination.

Abbreviations: AUC = area under curve; CI = confidence Interval; CT = *Chlamydia trachomatis*; F = female; M = male; n = number; Neg = negative; NNI = number needed to invite; NNS = number needed to screen; NR = not reported; Pos = positive.

Appendix C4. Quality Rating of Observational Study

Author, year	Did the study attempt to enroll all patients meeting inclusion criteria, or a random sample?	Were the groups comparable at baseline on key prognostic factors?	Did the study use accurate methods for ascertaining exposures and potential confounders?	Were outcome assessors and/or data analysts blinded to the exposure being studied?	Did the study maintain comparable groups?	Did the study perform appropriate statistical analyses on potential confounders?	Is there important differential or overall high loss to followup?	Were outcomes prespecified, defined, and ascertained using accurate methods?	Quality rating
Gotz et al, 2006[29]	Yes	Yes	Unclear	No	Yes	Yes	No	Yes	Good

Appendix C5. Diagnostic Accuracy Studies of Gonorrhea Tests

Study, year	Screening test	Definition of a positive screening exam	Reference standard	Country, Setting, Prevalence	Population characteristics
Chernesky et al, 2005[31]	AGC Site: urethral swab, FCU	Positive result from ≥1 NAAT in both urethral swab and FCU; or 1 specimen positive on both NAATs	AC2 PTGC	Canada, U.S. STI clinics	Age (mean): 28.5 y 100% male 62.2% non-Hispanic black, 24.6% white
Gaydos et al, 2013[36]	Xpert Site: self-collected vaginal, cervix, female FCU, male FCU	Positive result from at least 1 of the 2 reference NAATs	AC2 PTGC	U.S. STI clinics	Age: ≥14 y (range or mean NR) 45% male (full sample, asymptomatic information NR separately) Race: NR
Stewart et al, 2012[35]	AC2 Site: endocervical, self-collected vaginal	Positive culture with biochemical confirmation or positive result from 1 NAAT confirmed by second NAAT	Culture Aptima GC	United Kingdom Sexual health clinic Prevalence: NR	Age (mean): 25 y 100% female Ethnicity: 80% white, 9% black, 7% mixed, 4% other
Taylor et al, 2012[32]	c4800 Site: FCU AC2, CT/GC C^x Site: FCU, urethral swab	Positive result from ≥2 NAATs with different target regions in urethral swab and/or FCU	AC2 CT/GC Q^x	U.S. Obstetrics/gynecology, family planning, and STI clinics Prevalence: ≥1%	Age: 55% ≤30 y 100% male Race: 64.7% black, 32.9% white, 0.4% Asian, 0.4% American Indian/Alaskan Native, 0.1% Hawaiian/Pacific Islander, 1.3% other, 0.1% unknown Ethnicity: 82.7% non-Hispanic, 15.1% Hispanic, 2.2% unknown
Van Der Pol et al, 2012[33]	c4800, AC2, CT/GC Q^x Site: endocervical, FCU	Positive result from ≥2 NAATs with different target regions in endocervical swab and/or FCU; each NAAT was evaluated based on results of other 2 NAATS	AC2 CT/GC Q^x	U.S. Family planning, obstetrics/gynecology, and STI clinics Prevalence NR	Age: ≥14 y 100% female Race: 43.1% black, 48.4% white, 2.8% Asian/Pacific Islander, 5.7% other Ethnicity: 22.1% Hispanic
Van Der Pol et al, 2012[34]	GCQ, PTNG, AC2 Site: endocervical, female FCU, urethral swab, male FCU, all female sites, all male sites, overall	≥1 positive result from each reference NAAT; for assay comparison, positive result required from each of other 2 assays	AC2 PTNG	U.S. NG prevalence across sites (range): 1.4% to 19.2% in females; 4.8% to 40.5% in males	Age (range): 16 to 64 y 44% male Race: NR Note: 2.7% of females were pregnant

Study, year	Sample size Proportion with condition	Proportion unexaminable by screening test	Number of indeterminate results
Chernesky et al, 2005[31]	1322 enrolled 17.9% CT 13.8% NG	NR	NR
Gaydos et al, 2013[36]	2,270 asymptomatic 3.5% CT 0.7% NG	NR	0.25% (total sample) were invalid and unreadable
Stewart et al, 2012[35]	3973 enrolled 2.5% with NG	0.8%	None
Taylor et al, 2012[32]	768 enrolled 16.4% CT 9.2% NG	2.9%	NR
Van Der Pol et al, 2012[33]	4479 enrolled 6.3% CT 1.5% NG	3.6% of enrolled; 16.4% for primary analysis of particular specimen type	NR

Study, year	Eligibility Criteria
Chernesky et al, 2005[31]	Men ages 15 to 77 y. Excluded if could not concurrently provide all samples, had urinated within 1 hour, had taken antibiotics in the last 21 days, or if they could not provide informed consent.
Gaydos et al, 2013[36]	Age ≥14 y, sexually active in the last 6 months, and attending a participating clinic. Excluded if enrolled in previous trial, received antimicrobial therapy within 21 days of study, or history of hysterectomy.
Stewart et al, 2012[35]	Women age ≥16 y presenting to study clinic for a new visit. Excluded if used antibiotics in the last 28 days, were unable or unwilling to perform self-taken swab or have the standard examination and swabs performed by clinicians.
Taylor et al, 2012[32]	Men age ≥14 y. Excluded if they had been previously enrolled in the study or used antimicrobials effective against CT or NG in the last 21 days.
Van Der Pol et al, 2012[33]	Women age ≥14 y who were eligible for routine CT/NG screening as per standard practice at each enrollment site. Excluded if they had been previously enrolled, used antimicrobial agents active against CT or NG in last 21 days, used Faplense (a vaginal lubricant) within past 3 days, or had a

Appendix C5. Diagnostic Accuracy Studies of Gonorrhea Tests

Study, year	Eligibility Criteria	Sample size Proportion with condition	Proportion unexaminable by screening test	Number of indeterminate results
	history of hysterectomy or contraindication to Pap test/cervical sampling.			
Van Der Pol et al, 2012[34]	Men and women ages 16 to 64 y who presented with urogenital symptoms or were being screened for CT and NG. Excluded if they had urinated within 1 hour of specimen collection, used antibiotics within last 21 days, had prior study enrollment, failed to provide consent, or were younger than the age required by the sites' IRB.	1846 enrolled 6.5% of females with NG 14.5% of males with NG	4.2% 12% of males had only 2 urethral swabs collected, rather than 3	21 indeterminate from PTNG; 9/21 resolved negative with repeat testing, 12 remained indeterminate. All were negative by GCQ and AC2.

Study, year	Screening test	Proportion with reference standard & included in analysis	True positives	False positives	False negatives	True negatives	Proportion unexaminable by screening test	Sensitivity (95% CI)	Specificity (95% CI)
Chernesky et al, 2005[31]	AGC Site: urethral swab	100%	110	21	0	710		100.0% (71.5 to 100) Calculated CI: 96.7 to 100	97.1% (95.6 to 98.2)
	AGC Site: FCU		100	4	10	730		90.9% (58.7 to 99.8) Calculated CI: 83.9 to 95.6	99.5% (98.6 to 99.9)
Gaydos et al, 2013[36]	Xpert Site: self-collected vaginal	99.6%	12	1	0	1119		100% (77.9 to 100)	99.9% (99.5 to 100)
	Xpert Site: cervix		12	0	0	1116		100% (77.9 to 100)	100% (99.7 to 100)
	Xpert Site: female FCU		11	1	1	1123		91.7% (61.5 to 99.8)	99.9% (99.5 to 100)
	Xpert Site: male FCU		5	1	0	1126		100% (54.9 to 100)	99.9% (99.5 to 100)
Stewart et al, 2012[35]	AC2 Site: endocervical	97%	36	0	4	2194		90.0% (77.0 to 96.0)	100.0% (99.8 to 100.0)*
	AC2 Site: self-collected vaginal		39	0	1	2194		98.0% (87.0 to 100.0)	100.0% (99.8 to 100.0)*
Taylor et al, 2012[32]	c4800 Site: FCU	97.1%	7	0	0	465		100.0% (64.6 to 100.0) Calculated CI: 58.9 to 100	100.0% (99.2 to 100.0)
	AC2 Site: FCU		7	0	0	465		100.0% (64.6 to 100.0) Calculated CI: 58.9 to 100	100.0% (99.2 to 100.0)
	AC2 Site: urethral swab		7	0	0	465		100.0% (64.6 to 100.0) Calculated CI: 58.9 to 100	100.0% (99.2 to 100.0)
	CT/GC Q^X Site: FCU		7	1	0	464		100.0% (64.6 to 100.0) Calculated CI: 58.9 to 100	99.8% (98.8 to 100.0)
	CT/GC Q^X Site: urethral swab		7	0	0	465		100.0% (64.6 to 100.0) Calculated CI: 58.9 to 100	100.0% (99.2 to 100.0)
Van Der Pol et al, 2012[33]	c4800 Site: endocervical	96.4%	22	0	1	2246		95.7% (79.0 to 99.2)	100.0% (99.8 to 100.0)
	c4800 Site: FCU		23	1	0	2255		100.0% (85.7 to 100.0)	100.0% (99.7 to 100.0)
	AC2 Site: endocervical		23	0	0	2266		100.0% (85.7 to 100.0)	100.0% (99.8 to 100.0)
	AC2 Site: FCU		22	1	1	2268		95.7% (79.0 to 99.2)	100.0% (99.8 to 100.0)
	CT/GC Q^X Site: endocervical		21	4	2	2241		91.3% (73.2 to 97.6)	99.8% (99.5 to 99.9)
	CT/GC Q^X Site: FCU		23	3	0	2246		100.0% (85.7 to 100.0)	99.9% (99.6 to 100.0)

Appendix C5. Diagnostic Accuracy Studies of Gonorrhea Tests

Study, year	Screening test	Proportion with reference standard & included in analysis	True positives	False positives	False negatives	True negatives	Sensitivity (95% CI)	Specificity (95% CI)
Van Der Pol et al, 2012[34]	GCQ Site: endocervical	95.8%	26	2	1	421	96.3% (81.0 to 99.9)	99.5% (98.3 to 99.9)
	GCQ Site: female FCU		27	2	0	421	100.0% (87.2 to 100.0)	99.5% (98.3 to 99.9)
	GCQ Site: urethral swab		12	4	0	492	100.0% (73.5 to 100.0)	99.2% (97.9 to 99.8)
	GCQ Site: male FCU		12	4	0	501	100.0% (73.5 to 100.0%)	99.2% (98.0 to 99.8%)
	GCQ All female sites		106	13	2	1678	98.1% (93.5 to 99.8)	99.2% (98.7 to 99.6)
	GCQ All male sites		36	12	0	1494	100.0% (90.3 to 100.0)	99.2% (98.6 to 99.6)
	GCQ Overall		142	25	2	3172	98.6% (95.1 to 99.8)	99.2% (98.8 to 99.5)
	PTNG Site: endocervical		26	3	2	407	92.9% (76.5 to 99.1)	99.3% (97.9 to 99.8)
	PTNG Site: female FCU		23	2	5	414	82.1% (63.1 to 93.9)	99.5% (98.3 to 99.9)
	PTNG Site: urethral swab		12	0	0	480	100.0% (73.5 to 100.0)	100.0% (99.2 to 100.0)
	PTNG Site: male FCU		12	1	1	497	92.3% (64.0 to 99.8)	99.8% (98.9 to 100.0)
	PTNG All female sites		49	5	7	821	87.5% (75.9 to 94.8)	99.4% (98.6 to 99.8)
	PTNG All male sites		24	1	1	977	96.0% (79.6 to 99.9)	99.9% (99.4 to 100.0)
	PTNG Overall		73	6	8	1798	90.1% (81.5 to 95.6)	99.7% (99.3 to 99.9)
	AC2 Site: endocervical		27	2	1	418	96.4% (81.7 to 99.9)	99.5% (98.3 to 99.9)
	AC2 Site: female FCU		22	0	6	422	78.6% (59.0 to 91.7)	100.0% (99.1 to 100.0)
	AC2 Site: urethral swab		11	4	0	469	100.0% (71.5 to 100.0)	99.2% (97.8 to 99.8)
	AC2 Site: male FCU		12	3	0	502	100.0% (73.5 to 100.0)	99.4% (98.3 to 99.9)
	AC2 All female sites		49	2	7	840	87.5% (75.9 to 94.8)	99.8% (99.1 to 100.0)
	AC2 All male sites		23	7	0	971	100.0% (85.2 to 100.0)	99.3% (98.5 to 99.7)
	AC2 Overall		72	9	7	1811	91.1% (82.6 to 96.4)	99.5% (99.1 to 99.8)

Study, year	Screening test	Positive likelihood ratio (95% CI)	Negative likelihood ratio (95% CI)	Positive predictive value (95% CI)	Negative predictive value (95% CI)	Sponsor	Quality rating
Chernesky et al, 2005[31]	AGC Site: urethral swab	34.8 (22.8 to 53.1)*	0.00*	84.0% (76.5 to 89.8)*	100% (99.5 to 100.0)*	NR	Fair
	AGC Site: FCU	166.8 (62.7 to 444.1)*	0.09 (0.05 to 0.17)*	96.2% (90.4 to 98.9)*	98.7% (97.5 to 99.4)*		

Appendix C5. Diagnostic Accuracy Studies of Gonorrhea Tests

Study, year	Screening test	Positive likelihood ratio (95% CI)	Negative likelihood ratio (95% CI)	Positive predictive value (95% CI)	Negative predictive value (95% CI)	Sponsor	Quality rating
Gaydos et al, 2013[36]	Xpert Site: self-collected vaginal	1120.0 (157.90 to 7944.29)*	0.00*	92.3% (63.9 to 98.7)	100% (99.7 to 100)	Cepheid, grant from National Insitute of Biomedical Imaging and Bioengineering	Fair
	Xpert Site: cervix	Unable to calculate	0.00*	100.0% (73.4 to 100)	100.0% (99.7 to 100)		
	Xpert Site: female FCU	1030.3 (144.2 to 7362.7)*	0.08 (0.01 to 0.54)*	91.7% (61.5 to 98.6)	99.9% (99.5 to 99.9)		
	Xpert Site: male FCU	1127.0 (158.9 to 7993.9)*	0.00*	83.3% (36.1 to 97.2)	100.0% (99.7 to 100)		
Stewart et al, 2012[35]	AC2 Site: endocervical	Unable to calculate	0.10 (0.04 to 0.25)*	100.0% (90.2 to 100.0)*	99.8% (99.5 to 100.0)*	None reported (GenProbe provided supplies)	Good
	AC2 Site: self-collected vaginal	Unable to calculate	0.03 (0.00 to 0.17)*	100.0% (90.9 to 100.0)*	100.0% (99.8 to 100.0)*		
Taylor et al, 2012[32]	c4800 Site: FCU	Unable to calculate	0.00*	100% (58.9 to 100.0)*	100.0% (99.2 to 100.0)*	Roche Molecular Systems	Fair
	AC2 Site: FCU	Unable to calculate	0.00*	100% (58.9 to 100.0)*	100.0% (99.2 to 100.0)*		
	AC2 Site: urethral swab	Unable to calculate	0.00*	100% (58.9 to 100.0)*	100.0% (99.2 to 100.0)*		
	CT/GC Q[x] Site: FCU	465.0 (65.6 to 3294.2)*	0.00*	87.5% (47.4 to 97.9)*	100.0% (99.2 to 100.0)*		
	CT/GC Q[x] Site: urethral swab	Unable to calculate	0.00*	100% (58.9 to 100.0)*	100.0% (99.2 to 100.0)*		
Van Der Pol et al, 2012[33]	c4800 Site: endocervical	Unable to calculate	0.04 (0.01 to 0.30)*	100.0% (84.4 to 100.0)*†	100.0% (99.8 to 100.0)*	Roche Molecular Systems	Fair
	c4800 Site: FCU	2256.0 (317.9 to 16009.1)*	0.00*	95.8% (78.8 to 99.3)*	100.0% (99.8 to 100.0)*		
	AC2 Site: endocervical	Unable to calculate	0.00*	100.0% (85.1 to 100.0)	100.0% (99.8 to 100.0)*		
	AC2 Site: FCU	2170.4 (305.3 to 15431.2)*	0.04 (0.01 to 0.30)*	95.7% (78.0 to 99.3)*	100.0% (99.8 to 100.0)*		
	CT/GC Q[x] Site: endocervical	512.5 (190.9 to 1375.3)*	0.09 (0.02 to 0.33)*	84.0% (63.9 to 95.4)*	99.9% (99.7 to 100.0)*		
	CT/GC Q[x] Site: FCU	749.7 (242.0 to 2322.7)*	0.00*	88.5% (69.8 to 97.4)*	100.0% (99.8 to 100.0)*		
Van Der Pol et al, 2012[34]	GCQ Site: endocervical	203.7 (51.0 to 813.3)*	0.04 (0.01 to 0.25)*	92.9% (76.5 to 98.9)*	99.8% (98.7 to 100.0)*	BD Diagnostics	Fair
	GCQ Site: female FCU	211.5 (53.1 to 842.9)*	0.00*	93.1% (77.2 to 99.0)*	100.0% (99.1 to 100.0)*		
	GCQ Site: urethral swab	124.0 (46.7 to 329.1)*	0.00*	75.0% (47.6 to 92.6)*	100.0% (99.3 to 100.0)*		
	GCQ Site: male FCU	126.3 (47.6 to 335.1)*	0.00*	75.0% (47.6 to 92.6)*	100.0% (99.3 to 100.0)*		
	GCQ All female sites	127.7 (74.2 to 219.6)*	0.02 (0.00 to 0.07)*	89.1% (82.0 to 94.1)*	99.9% (99.6 to 100.0)*		
	GCQ All male sites	125.5 (71.4 to 220.5)*	0.00*	75.0% (60.4 to 86.4)*	100.0% (99.8 to 100.0)*		
	GCQ Overall	126.1 (85.3 to 186.4)*	0.01 (0.00 to 0.06)*	85.0% (78.7 to 90.1)*	99.9% (99.8 to 100.0)*		
	PTNG Site: endocervical	126.9 (40.9 to 393.7)*	0.07 (0.02 to 0.27)*	89.7% (72.6 to 97.7)*	99.5% (98.2 to 99.9)*		

Appendix C5. Diagnostic Accuracy Studies of Gonorrhea Tests

Study, year	Screening test	Positive likelihood ratio (95% CI)	Negative likelihood ratio (95% CI)	Positive predictive value (95% CI)	Negative predictive value (95% CI)	Sponsor	Quality rating
	PTNG Site: female FCU	170.9 (42.4 to 688.3)*	0.18 (0.08 to 0.40)*	92.0% (73.9 to 98.8)*	98.8% (97.2 to 99.6)*		
	PTNG Site: urethral swab	Unable to calculate	0.00*	100.0% (73.4 to 100.0)*	100.0% (99.2 to 100.0)*		
	PTNG Site: male FCU	459.7 (64.5 to 3277.6)*	0.08 (0.01 to 0.51)*	92.3% (63.9 to 98.7)*	99.8% (98.9 to 100.0)*		
	PTNG All female sites	144.6 (60.0 to 348.3)*	0.13 (0.06 to 0.25)*	90.7% (79.7 to 96.9)*	99.2% (98.3 to 99.7)*		
	PTNG All male sites	938.9 (132.2 to 6669.6)*	0.04 (0.01 to 0.27)*	96.0% (79.6 to 99.3)*	99.9% (99.4 to 100.0)*		
	PTNG Overall	271.0 (121.5 to 604.3)	0.10 (0.05 to 0.19)*	92.4% (84.2 to 97.1)*	99.6% (99.1 to 99.8)*		
	AC2 Site: endocervical	202.5 (50.7 to 808.5)*	0.04 (0.01 to 0.25)*	93.1% (77.2 to 99.0)*	99.8% (98.7 to 100.0)*		
	AC2 Site: female FCU	Unable to calculate	0.21 (0.11 to 0.44)*	100.0% (84.4 to 100.0)*	98.6% (97.0 to 99.5)*		
	AC2 Site: urethral swab	118.3 (44.6 to 313.8)*	0.00*	73.3% (44.9 to 92.1)*	100.0% (99.2 to 100.0)*		
	AC2 Site: male FCU	168.3 (54.5 to 520.2)*	0.00*	80.0% (51.9 to 95.4)*	100.0% (99.3 to 100.0)*		
	AC2 All female sites	368.4 (92.0 to 1475.8)*	0.13 (0.06 to 0.25)*	96.1% (86.5 to 99.4)*	99.2% (98.3 to 99.7)*		
	AC2 All male sites	139.7 (66.8 to 292.3)*	0.00*	76.7% (57.7 to 90.0)*	100.0% (99.6 to 100.0)*		
	AC2 Overall	184.3 (95.7 to 354.9)*	0.09 (0.04 to 0.18)*	88.9% (80.0 to 94.8)*	99.6% (99.2 to 99.8)*		

* Calculated.

† Authors estimate PPV = 93.8% to 99.9% (based on hypothetical prevalence range of 1% to 50%).

Abbreviations: AC2 = Aptima Combo 2; AGC = Aptima NG test; BD = Becton Dickinson; c4800= cobas 4800 CT and NG test; CI = confidence interval; CT = *Chlamydia trachomatis*; CT/GC Q^x = BD ProbeTec CT and NG Q^x amplified DNA assay; FCU = first-catch urine; GCQ = BD ProbeTec NG Q^x amplified DNA assay on Viper system; IRB = institutional review board; NAAT = nucleic acid amplification test; NG = *Neisseria gonorrhea*; NR = not reported; PPV = positive predictive value; PTGC = BD ProbeTec ET for CT and NG; PTNG = BD ProbeTec ET NG amplified DNA assay; STI = sexually transmited infection.

Appendix C6. Diagnostic Accuracy Studies of Chlamydia Tests

Study, year	Screening test(s)	Definition of a positive screening exam	Reference standard(s)	Country Setting Prevalence
NAATs vs. NAATs				
Chernesky et al, 2005[31]	ACT Site: urethral swab, FCU	Positive result from at least 1 NAAT in both urethral swab and FCU; or one specimen positive on both NAATs	AC2 PTGC	Canada, U.S. STI clinics
Gaydos et al, 2013[36]	Xpert Site: self-collected vaginal, cervix, female FCU, male FCU	Positive result from at least 1 of the reference NAATs	AC2 PTGC	U.S. STI clinics
Schachter et al, 2003[37]	ACT, Amplicor Site: FCU, cervix, clinician-collected vaginal, self-collected vaginal	Agreement between positive results with vaginal swab and cervical swab or FCU	Culture	U.S., Canada Family planning, obstetrics/gynecology, and STI clinics CT prevalence across sites: 5.4% to 10.2% by culture
Schoeman et al, 2012[40]	AC2 Site: endocervix, self-collected vaginal	Positive result from 1 NAAT confirmed by second NAAT	Aptima CT	United Kingdom Sexual health clinic Prevalence: NR
Shrier et al, 2004[38]	Amplicor Site: endocervix, FCU, clinician-collected vaginal, self-collected vaginal	1 positive culture or 2 positive nonculture tests or 1 positive nonculture test confirmed by nested PCR	Culture Amplicor Abbot LCx assay	U.S. University medical center and children's hospital 21.6% positive for CT at any site
Taylor et al, 2012[32]	c4800 Site: FCU AC2, CT/GC Q[x] Site: FCU, urethral swab	Positive result from ≥2 NAATs with different target regions in urethral swab and/or FCU	AC2 CT/GC Q[x]	U.S. Obstetrics/gynecology, family planning, and STI clinics Prevalence ≥1%
Taylor et al, 2011[39]	CTQ, PTCT, AC2 Site: endocervical, female FCU, urethral swab, male FCU, all female sites, all male sites	≥1 positive result from each reference NAAT; for assay comparison, positive result required from each of other 2 assays	AC2 PTCT	U.S. Family planning, obstetrics/gynecology, and STI clinics CT prevalence across sites: 11.6% in females, 21.4% in males
Van Der Pol et al, 2012[33]	c4800, AC2, CT/GC Q[x] Site: endocervical, FCU	Positive result from ≥2 NAATs with different target regions in endocervical swab and/or FCU; each NAAT was evaluated based on results of other 2 NAATs	AC2 CT/GC Q[x]	U.S. Family planning, obstetrics/gynecology, and STI clinics Prevalence NR

Study, year	Population Characteristics	Eligibility Criteria	Sample size Proportion with condition
NAATs vs. NAATs			
Chernesky et al, 2005[31]	Age (mean): 28.5 y 100% male 62.2% non-Hispanic black, 24.6% white	Men ages 15 to 77 y. Excluded if they could not concurrently provide all samples, had urinated within 1 hour, had taken antibiotics in the last 21 days, or if they could not provide informed consent.	1322 enrolled 17.9% CT 13.8% NG
Gaydos et al, 2013[36]	Age: ≥14 y (range or mean NR) 45% male (full sample, asymptomatic information NR separately) Race: NR	Age ≥14 y, sexually active in the last 6 months, and attending a participating clinic. Excluded if enrolled in previous trial, received antimicrobial therapy within 21 days of study, or history of hysterectomy.	2,270 asymptomatic 3.5% CT 0.7% NG

Appendix C6. Diagnostic Accuracy Studies of Chlamydia Tests

Study, year	Population Characteristics	Eligibility Criteria	Sample size Proportion with condition
Schachter et al, 2003[37]	Age (range): 16 to 25 y 100% female Race: NR	Females ages 16 to 25 y who were not pregnant and attending a study clinic for routine exam or birth control advice. Excluded if they had been treated with antibiotics within the last 30 days, were attending the clinic because of symptoms, or had a male partner treated for genital symptoms.	2517 tested 9.6% of women with CT by culture of 1 specimen
Schoeman et al, 2012[40]	Age (mean): 25 y 100% female Ethnicity: 80% white, 9% black, 7% mixed, 4% other	Women age ≥16 y presenting to study clinic for a new visit. Excluded if used antibiotics in the preceding 28 days, were unable or unwilling to perform self-taken swab, or have the standard exam and swabs performed by clinicians.	3973 enrolled 10.3% with CT
Shrier et al, 2004[38]	Age (mean): 19 y 100% female 22% history of CT Median time since previous CT infection: 539 days (range, 43 to 2738) 8% with history of other STI	Females ages 16 to 25 y who had ever had sexual intercourse, did not report symptoms of an STI, and were being seen at clinic for routine gynecologic care. Excluded if they were pregnant, had taken antibiotics in the previous 21 days, were diagnosed with CT in the previous 6 weeks, or had sexual contact with a partner diagnosed with an STI.	139 eligible 126 analyzed 21.6% CT 2% NG or trichomoniasis (1 participant had CT and NG)
Taylor et al, 2012[32]	Age: 55% ≤30 y 100% male Race: 64.7% black, 32.9% white, 0.4% Asian, 0.4% American Indian/Alaskan Native, 0.1% Hawaiian/Pacific Islander, 1.3% other, 0.1% unknown Ethnicity: 82.7% non-Hispanic, 15.1% Hispanic, 2.2% unknown ethnicity	Men age ≥14 y. Excluded if they had been previously enrolled in the study or used antimicrobials effective against CT or NG in the preceding 21 days.	768 enrolled 16.4% CT 9.2% NG
Taylor et al, 2011[39]	Age (range): 17 to 64 y 32% male Race: NR Note: 2.7% of females were pregnant	Men and women ages 17 to 64 y who presented with urogenital symptoms or were being screened for CT and NG. Excluded if they had taken antibiotics in the previous 21 days, urinated in the previous hour, had sample collection issues, did not provide informed consent, or were younger than the age required by the site's IRB.	1538 enrolled 11.6% of females with CT 21.4% of males with CT
Van Der Pol et al, 2012[33]	Age: ≥14 y 100% female 43.1% black, 48.4% white, 22.1% Hispanic, 2.8% Asian/Pacific Islander, 5.7% other	Women age ≥14 y who were eligible for routine CT/NG screening as per standard practice at each enrollment site. Excluded if they had been previously enrolled, used antimicrobial agents active against CT or NG in preceding 21 days, used Raplense, a vaginal lubricant, within the past 3 days, or had a history of hysterectomy or contraindication to Pap test/cervical sampling.	4479 enrolled 6.3% CT 1.5% NG

Appendix C6. Diagnostic Accuracy Studies of Chlamydia Tests

NAATs vs. NAATs

Study, year	Screening test(s)	Proportion unexaminable by screening test	Number of indeterminate results	Proportion who underwent reference standard and included in analysis	True positives	False positives	False negatives	True negatives	Sensitivity (95% CI)
Chernesky et al, 2005[31]	ACT Site: urethral swab	NR	NR	100%	94	16	1	634	98.9% (94.3 to 100)
	Site: FCU				94	19	1	638	98.9% (94.3 to 100)
Gaydos et al, 2013[36]	Xpert Site: self-collected vaginal	NR	0.25% (total sample) were invalid and unreadable	99.6%	48	7	1	1076	98.0% (89.1 to 99.9)
	Site: cervix				46	6	2	1074	95.8% (85.7 to 99.5)
	Site: female FCU				49	2	2	1083	96.1% (86.5 to 99.5)
	Site: male FCU				29	1	0	1102	100% (90.2 to 100)
Schachter et al, 2003[37]	ACT Site: FCU	Not reported	Not reported	Unclear	86*	7	33*	1265*	72.0%
	Site: cervix				106*	10	13*	1262*	89.1%
	Site: clinician-collected vaginal				107*	9	12*	1263*	89.9%
	Site: self-collected vaginal				111*	6	8*	1266*	93.3%
	Amplicor Site: FCU				63*	5	12*	501*	84.0%
	Site: cervix				68*	3	7*	503*	90.7%
	Site: clinician-collected vaginal				70*	6	5*	500*	93.3%
	Site: self-collected vaginal				68*	5	7*	501*	90.7%
Schoeman et al, 2012[40]	AC2 Site: endocervix	0.7%	4	97.3%	163	0	20	2050	89.0% (84.0 to 93.0)
	Site: self-collected vaginal				178	1	5	2049	97.0% (94.0 to 99.0)
Shrier et al, 2004[38]	Amplicor Site: endocervix	1 participant excluded because no samples were collected by physician	None reported; 8 participants had a single positive result that needed confirmation by nested PCR	90.6% (analysis only included eligible participants with results on all tests)	14	0	13	99	51.9% (32.0 to 71.3)
	Site: FCU				12	0	15	99	44.4% (26.9 to 63.6)
	clinician-collected vaginal				15	0	12	99	55.6% (36.4 to 73.1)
	self-collected vaginal				14	1	13	98	51.9% (32.0 to 71.3)
Taylor et al, 2012[32]	c4800 Site: FCU	2.9%	NR	97.1%	51	2	1	418	98.1% (89.9 to 99.7)
	AC2 Site: FCU				50	4	1	417	98.0% (89.7 to 99.7)
	Site: urethral swab				48	5	3	416	94.1% (84.1 to 98.0)
	CT/GC Q^x Site: FCU				50	2	2	418	96.2% (87.0 to 98.9)
	Site: urethral swab				45	1	7	419	86.5% (74.7 to 93.3)

Appendix C6. Diagnostic Accuracy Studies of Chlamydia Tests

Study, year	Screening test(s)	Proportion unexaminable by screening test	Number of indeterminate results	Proportion who underwent reference standard and included in analysis	True positives	False positives	False negatives	True negatives	Sensitivity (95% CI)
Taylor et al, 2011[39]	CTQ Site: endocervical	4.7%; 13% of men had only 2 urethral swabs collected rather than 3	19 unable to calculate from PTCT; 7/19 resolved negative All 19 were negative by CTQ and AC2	95.3%	53	8	4	385	93.0% (83.0 to 98.1)
	Site: female FCU				54	2	3	391	94.7% (85.4 to 98.9)
	Site: urethral swab				31	2	4	178	88.6% (73.3 to 96.8)
	Site: Male FCU				35	2	0	178	100.0% (90.0 to 100.0)
	All female sites				216	12	12	1559	94.7% (91.0 to 97.3)
	All male sites				101	6	4	534	96.2% (90.5 to 99.0)
	PTCT Site: endocervical				51	0	8	379	86.4% (75.0 to 94.0)
	Site: female FCU				53	1	6	384	89.8% (79.2 to 96.2)
	Site: urethral swab				31	2	5	173	86.1% (70.5 to 95.3)
	Site: male FCU				35	1	1	173	97.2% (85.5 to 99.9)
	All female sites				104	1	14	763	88.1% (80.9 to 93.4)
	All male sites				66	3	6	346	91.7% (82.7 to 96.9%)
	AC2 Site: endocervical				52	4	4	389	92.9% (82.7 to 98.0)
	Site: female FCU				55	2	1	392	98.2% (90.4 to 100.0)
	Site: urethral swab				30	2	3	166	90.9% (75.7 to 98.1)
	Site: male FCU				35	0	1	179	97.2% (85.5 to 99.9)
	All female sites				107	6	5	781	95.5% (89.9 to 98.5)
	All male sites				65	2	4	345	94.2% (85.8 to 98.4)
Van Der Pol et al, 2012[33]	c4830 Site: endocervical	3.6% of enrolled; 16.4% for primary analysis of particular specimen type	NR	96.4%	94	1	11	2163	89.5% (82.2 to 94.0)
	Site: FCU				98	4	12	2165	89.1% (81.9 to 93.6)
	AC2 Site: endocervical				101	12	3	2173	97.1% (91.9 to 99.0)
	Site: FCU				98	5	8	2181	92.5% (85.8 to 96.1)
	CT/GC Q^x Site: endocervical				102	7	4	2155	96.2% (90.7 to 98.5)
	Site: FCU				101	6	4	2161	96.2% (90.6 to 98.5)

Study, year	Screening test(s)	Specificity (95% CI)	Positive likelihood ratio (95% CI)	Negative likelihood ratio (95% CI)	Positive predictive value (95% CI)	Negative predictive value (95% CI)	Sponsor	Quality rating
NAATs vs. NAATs								
Chernesky et al, 2005[31]	ACT Site urethral swab	97.5% (96.0 to 98.6)	40.2 (24.8 to 65.3)*	0.01 (0.00 to 0.08)*	85.5% (77.5 to 91.5)*	99.8% (99.1 to 100)*	NR	Fair
	ACT Site: FCU	98.0% (96.6 to 98.9)	34.2 (22.0 to 53.3)*	0.01 (0 to 0.08)*	83.2% (75 to 89.6)*	99.8% (99.1 to 100)*		
Gaydos et al, 2013[36]	Xpert Site: self-collected vaginal	97.1% (95.5 to 98.3)*	151.6 (72.3 to 317.5)*	0.02 (0.00 to 0.14)*	87.3% (75.5 to 94.7)	99.9% (99.5 to 99.9)	Cepheid, grant from National Institute of Biomedical Imaging and Bioengineering	Fair
	Site: cervix	98.4% (98.7 to 99.7)	172.5 (77.5 to 383.9)*	0.04 (0.01 to 0.16)*	88.5% (76.5 to 95.6)	99.8% (99.3 to 99.7)		
	Site: female FCU	98.4% (98.8 to 99.8)*	521.2 (130.4 to 2083.8)*	0.04 (0.01 to 0.15)*	96.1% (86.5 to 99.4)	99.8% (99.3 to 99.9)		
	Site: male FCU	98.8% (99.3 to 100); 98.9% (99.5 to 100)	1103.0 (155.5 to 7823.6)*	0.00*	96.7% (82.7 to 99.4)	100% (99.6 to 100)		

Appendix C6. Diagnostic Accuracy Studies of Chlamydia Tests

Study, year	Screening test(s)	Specificity (95% CI)	Positive likelihood ratio (95% CI)	Negative likelihood ratio (95% CI)	Positive predictive value (95% CI)	Negative predictive value (95% CI)	Sponsor	Quality rating
Schachter et al, 2003[37]	ACT Site: FCU	99.5%	131.3 (62.2 to 277.2)*	0.28 (0.21 to 0.37)*	92.5% (85.1 to 96.9)*	97.5% (96.5 to 98.2)*	Roche Molecular Systems; Abbott Laboratories; GenProbe, Inc; CDC	Fair
	Site: cervix	99.3%	113.3 (60.9 to 210.7)*	0.11 (0.07 to 0.18)*	91.4% (84.7 to 95.8)*	99.0% (98.3 to 99.5)*		
	Site: clinician-collected vaginal	99.4%	127.1 (66.1 to 244.4)*	0.10 (0.06 to 0.17)*	92.2% (85.8 to 96.4)*	99.1% (98.4 to 99.5)*		
	Site: self-collected vaginal	99.6%	197.8 (88.9 to 440.0)*	0.07 (0.03 to 0.13)*	94.9% (89.2 to 98.1)	99.4% (98.8 to 99.7)		
	Amplicor Site: FCU	99.0%	85.0 (35.3 to 204.5)	0.16 (0.10 to 0.27)*	92.7% (83.7 to 97.5)*	97.7% (96.0 to 98.8)*		
	Site: cervix	99.4%	152.9 (49.4 to 473.7)*	0.09 (0.05 to 0.19)*	95.8% (88.1 to 99.1)*	98.6% (97.2 to 99.4)*		
	Site: clinician-collected vaginal	98.8%	78.7 (35.5 to 174.7)*	0.07 (0.03 to 0.16)*	92.1% (83.6 to 97.0)*	99.0% (97.7 to 99.7)*		
	Site: self-collected vaginal	99.0%	91.8 (38.2 to 220.2)*	0.09 (0.05 to 0.19)*	93.2% (84.7 to 97.7)*	98.6% (97.2 to 99.4)*		
Schoeman et al, 2012[40]	AC2 Site: endocervix	100% (99.8 to 100.0)	Unable to calculate	0.11 (0.07 to 0.17)	100.0% (97.7 to 100.0)*	99.0% (98.5 to 99.4)*	None reported (GenProbe provided supplies)	Good
	Site: self-collected vaginal	99.9% (99.7 to 100.0)	1994.0 (281.0 to 14151.3)*	0.03 (0.01 to 0.06)*	99.4% (96.9 to 99.9)*	99.8% (99.4 to 99.9)*		
Shrier et al, 2004[38]	Amplicor Site: endocervix	100% (96.5 to 100)	Unable to calculate	0.48 (0.33 to 0.71)*	100% (77.0 to 100)	88.4% (81.1 to 93.6)	Roche Molecular Systems, Inc; CDC; NIMH, NIH	Good
	Site: FCU	100% (96.5 to 100)	0.56 (0.40 to 0.78)	Unable to calculate	100% (76.4 to 100)	86.8% (79.6 to 92.3)		
	Site: clinician-collected vaginal	100% (96.5 to 100)	Unable to calculate	0.44 (0.29 to 0.68)*	100% (78.7 to 100)	89.2% (82.4 to 94.0)		
	Site: self-collected vaginal	99.0% (95.0 to 100)	51.3 (7.1 to 373.2)*	0.49 (0.33 to 0.72)*	93.3% (69.8 to 99.7)	88.3% (81.0 to 93.5)		
Taylor et al, 2012[32]	c4800 Site: FCU	99.5% (98.3 to 99.9)	206.0 (51.7 to 821.3)*	0.02 (0.00 to 0.13)*	96.2% (87.0 to 99.4)*	99.8% (98.7 to 100.0)*	Roche Molecular Systems	Fair
	AC2 Site: FCU	99.0% (97.6 to 99.6)	103.2 (38.9 to 273.9)*	0.02 (0.00 to 0.14)*	92.6% (82.1 to 97.9)*	99.8% (98.7 to 100.0)*		
	Site: urethral swab	98.9% (97.3 to 99.5)	79.3 (33.1 to 189.9)*	0.06 (0.02 to 0.18)*	90.6% (79.3 to 96.8)*	99.3% (97.9 to 99.8)*		
	CT/GC Qx Site: FCU	99.5% (98.3 to 99.9)	201.9 (50.6 to 805.6)*	0.04 (0.01 to 0.15)*	96.2% (86.8 to 99.4)*	99.5% (98.3 to 99.9)*		
	Site: urethral swab	99.8% (98.7 to 100.0)	363.5 (51.2 to 2581.9)*	0.13 (0.07 to 0.27)*	97.8% (88.4 to 99.6)*	98.4% (96.6 to 99.3)*		
	CTQ Site: endocervix	98.0% (96.0 to 99.1)	45.7 (22.3 to 91.0)*	0.07 (0.03 to 0.18)	86.9% (75.8 to 94.2)*	99.0% (97.4 to 99.7)*		
	Site: female FCU	99.5% (98.2 to 99.9)	186.2 (46.7 to 742.7)*	0.05 (0.02 to 0.16)*	96.4% (87.7 to 99.5)*	99.2% (97.8 to 99.8)*		
	Site: urethral swab	98.9% (96.0 to 99.9)	79.7 (20.0 to 317.9)*	0.12 (0.05 to 0.29)*	93.9% (79.7 to 99.1)*	97.8% (94.5% to 99.4)*	BD Diagnostics	Fair
	Site: Male FCU	98.9% (96.0 to 99.9)	90.0 (22.7 to 357.1)*	0.00*	94.6% (81.8 to 99.2)*	100.0% (97.9 to 100.0)*		
	All female sites	99.2% (98.7 to 99.6)	124.0 (70.5 to 218.1)*	0.05 (0.03 to 0.09)	94.7% (91.0 to 97.3)*	99.2% (98.7 to 99.6)*		
	All male sites	98.8% (97.6 to 99.6%)	86.6 (39.0 to 192.0)*	0.04 (0.01 to 0.10)*	94.4% (88.2 to 97.9)*	99.3% (98.1 to 99.8)*		
	PTCT Site: endocervical	100.0% (99.0 to 100.0)	Unable to calculate	0.14 (0.07 to 0.26)*	100.0% (93.0 to 100.0)*	97.9% (96.0 to 99.1)*		
	Site: female FCU	99.7% (98.6 to 100.0)	345.9 (48.8 to 2453.7)*	0.10 (0.05 to 0.22)*	98.2% (90.1 to 99.7)*	98.5% (96.7 to 99.4)*		
	Site: urethral swab	98.9% (95.9 to 99.9)	75.4 (18.9 to 300.8)*	0.14 (0.06 to 0.32)*	93.9% (79.7 to 99.1)*	97.2% (93.6 to 99.1)*		
	Site: male FCU	99.4% (96.8 to 100.0)	169.2 (23.9 to 1195.2)*	0.03 (0.00 to 0.19)*	97.2% (85.4 to 99.5)*	99.4% (96.8 to 99.9)*		
	All female sites	99.9% (99.3 to 100.0)	673.4 (94.9 to 4779.6)*	0.12 (0.07 to 0.19)*	99.1% (94.8 to 99.8)*	98.2% (97.0 to 99.0)*		
	All male sites	99.1% (97.5 to 99.8)	106.6 (34.5 to 329.8)*	0.08 (0.04 to 0.18)*	95.6% (87.8 to 99.0)*	98.3% (96.3 to 99.4)*		
	AC2 Site: endocervical	99.0% (97.4 to 99.7)	91.2 (34.3 to 242.5)*	0.07 (0.03 to 0.19)*	92.9% (82.7 to 98.0)*	99.0% (97.4 to 99.7)*		
	Site: female FCU	99.5% (98.2 to 99.9)	193.5 (48.5 to 771.3)*	0.02 (0.00 to 0.13)*	96.5% (87.9 to 99.5)*	99.8% (98.6 to 100.0)*		

Appendix C6. Diagnostic Accuracy Studies of Chlamydia Tests

Study, year	Screening test(s)	Specificity (95% CI)	Positive likelihood ratio (95% CI)	Negative likelihood ratio (95% CI)	Positive predictive value (95% CI)	Negative predictive value (95% CI)	Sponsor	Quality rating
Taylor et al, 2011[39]	AC2 Site: urethral swab	98.8% (95.8 to 99.9)	76.4 (19.2 to 304.1)*	0.09 (0.03 to 0.27)*	93.8% (79.2 to 99.1)*	98.2% (94.9 to 99.6)*	BD Diagnostics	Fair
	Site: male FCU	100.0% (98.0 to 100.0)	Unable to calculate	0.03 (0.00 to 0.15)*	100.0% (89.9 to 100.0)*	99.4% (96.9 to 99.9)*		
	All female sites	99.2% (98.3 to 99.7)	125.3 (56.4 to 278.4)*	0.04 (0.02 to 0.11)*	94.7% (88.8 to 98.0)*	99.4% (98.5 to 99.8)*		
	All male sites	99.4% (97.9 to 99.9)	163.4 (41.0 to 651.7)*	0.06 (0.02 to 0.15)*	97.0% (89.6 to 99.6)*	98.9% (97.1 to 99.7)*		
Van Der Pol et al, 2012[33]	c4800 Site: endocervical	100.0% (99.7 to 100.0)	1937.3 (272.7 to 13762.3)*	0.10 (0.06 to 0.13)*	99.0% (94.3 to 99.8)* Note: authors estimate PPV of 77.3% to 99.7% (based on hypothetical prevalence range of 1% to 50%)	99.5% (99.1 to 99.8)*	Roche Molecular Systems	Fair
	Site: FCU	99.8% (99.5 to 99.9)	483.1 (181.1 to 1288.8)*	0.11 (0.06 to 0.19)*	96.1% (90.3 to 98.9)*	99.5% (99.0 to 99.7)*		
	AC2 Site: endocervical	99.5% (99.0 to 99.7)	176.8 (100.5 to 311.2)*	0.03 (0.01 to 0.09)*	89.4% (82.2 to 94.4)*	99.9% (99.6 to 100.0)*		
	Site: FCU	99.8% (99.5 to 99.9)	404.2 (168.1 to 971.8)*	0.08 (0.04 to 0.15)*	95.2% (89.0 to 98.4)*	99.6% (99.3 to 99.8)*		
	CT/GC Qx Site: endocervical	99.7% (99.3 to 99.8)	297.2 (141.7 to 623.3)*	0.04 (0.01 to 0.10)*	93.6% (87.2 to 97.3)*	99.8% (99.5 to 100.0)*		
	Site: FCU	99.7% (99.4 to 99.9)	347.4 (156.1 to 773.1)*	0.04 (0.01 to 0.10)*	94.4% (88.2 to 97.9)*	99.8% (99.5 to 100.0)*		

* Calculated.

Abbreviations: AC2 = Aptima Combo 2; ACT = Aptima Chlamydia trachomatis test; Amplicor = Roche cobas Amplicor test; BD = Becton Dickinson; c4800= Roche cobas 4800 CT and NG test; CDC = Centers for Disease Control and Prevention; CI = confidence interval; CT = Chlamydia trachomatis; CTQ = BD ProbeTec CT Qx amplified DNA assay on the Viper system; CT/GC Qx = BD ProbeTec CT and NG Qx amplified DNA assay; EIA = enzyme immunoassay; FCU = first-catch urine; IRB = institutional review board; NAAT = nucleic acid amplification test; NG = Neisseria gonorrhea; NIH = National Institutes of Health; NIMH = National Institute for Mental Health; NR = not reported; PCR = polymerase chain reaction; PT = ProbeTech; PTCT = BD ProbeTech ET CT amplified DNA assay; PTGC = BD ProbeTech ET amplified DNA assay for CT and NG; STI = sexually transmitted infection.

Appendix C7. Quality Ratings of Diagnostic Accuracy Studies

Study, year	Representative spectrum	Random or consecutive sample	Screening test adequately described	Screening cutoffs predefined	Credible reference standard	Reference standard applied to and analysis includes all patients, or a random subset	Same reference standard applied to all patients	Reference standard and screening examination interpreted independently	High rate of uninterpretable results or noncompliance with screening test	Analysis includes patients with uninterpretable results or noncompliance	Quality Rating
Chernesky et al, 2005[31]	Yes	Unclear	Yes	Yes	Yes	Yes	Yes	Unclear	Unclear	Unclear	Fair
Schacter et al, 2003[37]	Unclear	Unclear	Yes	Yes	Yes	Yes	Yes	Unclear	Unclear	Unclear	Fair
Schoeman et al, 2012[40]	Yes	Unclear	Yes	Yes	Yes	Yes	Yes	Unclear	No	Yes	Good
Shrier et al, 2004[38]	Yes	Unclear	Yes	Yes	Yes	Yes	Yes	Unclear	No	No	Fair
Stewart et al, 2012[35]	Yes	Unclear	Yes	Yes	Yes	Yes	Yes	Unclear	No	Yes	Good
Taylor et al, 2011[39]	Yes	Unclear	Yes	Yes	Yes	Yes	Yes	Unclear	No	Unclear	Fair
Taylor et al, 2012[32]	Yes	Unclear	Yes	Yes	Yes	Yes	Yes	Unclear	No	No	Fair
Van Der Pol et al, 2012[33]	Yes	Unclear	Yes	Yes	Yes	Yes	Yes	Unclear	No	Unclear	Fair
Van Der Pol et al, 2012[34]	Yes	Unclear	Yes	Yes	Yes	Yes	Yes	Unclear	No	Unclear	Fair
Gaydos et al, 2013[36]	Yes	Unclear	Yes	Yes	Yes	Yes	Yes	Unclear	No	Unclear	Fair

www.ingramcontent.com/pod-product-compliance
Lightning Source LLC
Chambersburg PA
CBHW080641180526
45168CB00008B/3264